MW01235048

Chakra Healing For Beginners

A Complete Guide to Awakening, Clearing, Unblocking and Balancing your Chakras and Your Life Through Guided meditations, Crystals, the Power of Affirmations and Yoga

Dr. Louise Lily Wain

Table of Contents

Introduction

Congratulations on downloading *Chakra Healing For Beginners* and thank you for doing so.

Just by taking the time to read this book and learn more about chakras already shows that you've taken a big step towards your spiritual path of acceptance of yourself and the world around you.

In this book, you will learn to understand that only you have the power and energy to heal yourself with the help of awakening all of your chakra points.

The universe is on your side, you can ask for guidance or help from the higher power when you feel lost on your path.

Don't be afraid to dive deeper into your inner wisdom in order to unlock the truth behind your existence and you being here.

In the following chapters, you will learn the basics of each chakra point, it's meaning, importance, how they affect a person both negatively and positively as well as many unique and easy ways to open a specific chakra point.

Many techniques such as guided meditations, yoga, affirmations, and even crystals can help balance out the chakras within your body, aligning them with your spirit and healing yourself.

With the help of this basic and easy understanding book, it is guaranteed that you will be able to balance out all of your seven chakras and heal the body, mind, and spirit.

There are plenty of books on this subject on the market, thanks again for choosing this one!

Every effort was made to ensure it is full of as much useful information as possible, please enjoy it!

Chapter 1: Chakra Introduction

In order to understand how to awaken your chakra point, you must first understand what and how important they are.

The flow of Ki is the energy within one's body, its purpose it so makes sure the body functions properly, it is also known as the 'life force'.

That flow of energy has specific concentrated areas within the body, and they are called chakras.

Chakras, or also known as cakra in some counties, are concentrated energy centers within the body that specialize in making sure that region or area works perfectly.

But many times, our negative thoughts and actions act like poison for the pure energies within our body, thus deactivating the proper flow of energy.

This is why many times a person suffers not only physically, but mentally, emotionally, and spiritually and it is all the cause of a blocked chakra.

The concept of chakras dates back almost hundreds of years ago, first originating in India within a text called Vedas, around 1500 B.C and 500 B.C.

This new discussion of the body being considered as a flow of energy evolved and traveled to different counties, and expanding its belief to numerous religions such as the Shri Jabala Darshana Upanishad, the Shandilya Upanishad, the Yoga-Shikka Upanishad, and countless of others.

But the chakra concept started to die down until a scholar by the name of Anodea Judith proceeded to write a book, 'Wheels of Life', which brought the concept not only back to life but all throughout Europe.

This caught people's belief and attention, causing more New Age writers to publish their books on the topic, spreading the belief all throughout eastern and western regions.

Chakras should not be viewed as just major energy centers within the body, in fact, chakras have their own colors, vibrational frequency, and most importantly, their own functions.

Not only they affect a person differently, but they can also affect each other.

The word 'chakra' originated from Sanskrit, it means 'wheel' or 'disk'.

Just like it's definition, chakras are a spinning wheel of energy and light within the body.

Together, they are identified as a blueprint for a healthy body by incorporating, taking in, and emanating the flow of Ki to help the body function properly and healthy.

However, due to our advanced mind, the chakras often get blocked and clogged, preventing the body from living a healthy life.

This energy is so pure that it often takes a lot of patience and consistency to be able to open the chakras and maintaining them in their healthy state.

Energy cannot be created or destroyed, in fact, energy's vibrations are the only thing that can be changed.

Everyone and everything vibrates on some level, if one is happy, the vibration of that being is very high, they are able to attract good things into their lives and influence the mood of others.

If one has a negative viewpoint on themselves and the world, then they have a low vibration.

Low vibration attracts low vibrational beings, things, and problems while high vibration attracts high vibrational things such as good people, trust, love, success, luck, and other good things into one's life.

Chakras have their own vibrations and oftentimes, those vibrations get polluted by every negative thought that crosses your mind and every bad action that one does.

Keeping an open mindset and having no negative thoughts is possible but very hard.

But with work and patience, you will be able to achieve it too.

When the mind is healthy, the body is healthy.

The energy goes where the thought goes meaning that if one constantly thinks negatively about an aspect of their body or their environment, then it will not make it disappear, but oftentimes, it can even make it worse.

Chakras are able to keep one balanced physically, mentally, and spiritually.

This healthy balance can change one's mindset and push them towards the direction of success.

It is very important to be able to maintain this healthy balance, awakening and balancing chakras can help the body achieve equilibrium.

Modern scientists were able to link many of the diseases that originated within one's body to the mind.

A mind is a powerful place, it is also in control of the heart which keeps the body alive and the energy which promotes the health of all the organs and tissues.

A wrong mindset can cause problems to emerge within the body.

There are countless minor chakras and only seven major chakras.

The major chakras can not only affect each other but also the minor chakras surrounding it.

When a major chakra is open, then the surrounding minor chakras are also open and in balance with each other.

An open major chakra can also be used to open and balance other major chakras and minor chakras. There are seven major chakras in total, each will be discussed in the following chapters.

The process of balancing and awakening chakras can be rather difficult, but it is not impossible.

Throughout life, almost everyone experiences an imbalance or a block in chakras due to the obstacles that life throws at us.

For example, having a blocked heart chakra can strongly affect one in terms of personal relationships with family or partners, one may also experience trust issues.

This is all because of past bad memories, or traumas that one hasn't let go of that makes a person the way that they are today.

By awakening chakras, one is learning to put everything that happened in the past behind them and move on with a new mindset and form new opportunities.

Chakras cannot be seen, but just because one doesn't see it, doesn't mean it's not there.

In fact, there are a lot of different reasons as to why a chakra is blocked and imbalanced.

They can be either physical or mental.

For example, if one doesn't provide the proper nutrients to the body from food, then the energy will reduce drastically and the flow of Ki may be corrupted.

There is energy within our bodies, but it is not as fresh and pure as one may think.

By eating healthy and taking in plenty of nutrients, you are able to not only promote the flow of energy within the body but also purify it and increase it.

Another example that relates to the mental state is the control of your feelings.

If you are unable to control your feelings such as frustration and anger or perhaps you are always lying to everyone, then the healthy flow of energy can be stopped.

Since each of the chakras works on a different level to keep the body and mind healthy, when more than one is imbalanced then they can often affect the physical world and the reality around you.

Just like a balanced chakra than can balance out other chakras, an imbalanced and unhealthy one is able to corrupt others too.

If many chakras are imbalanced then they can manifest into physical symptoms that are harder to correct, but not impossible.

Not only that, but the physical environment can also be affected as well as other people around you.

When one is often negative in terms of thinking and actions, they are able to cause other people pain and discomfort.

This affects the relationship between two people which can cause separation between friends, family, co-workers, or even lovers.

Each person has a different reason as to why their chakras are blocked, so spending some time to try to figure out which chakra it is and the cause of this chakra can help you further understand what you must to in order to heal that chakra and the body.

It is of great importance that these chakras remain healthy and well balanced due to their responsibility for many different aspects of one's lives.

For example, if the root chakra is in balance and healthy, one can be able to feel their foundation in this world which feels as if they are grounded within this reality.

However, when the root chakra doesn't work, then the person turns from a thinker and an achiever into a daydreamer who has a hard time to focus on anything.

Having an imbalanced root chakra won't be able to help you achieve your goals and the reason that you were born in this world at this time.

Another example is the throat chakra, if it works well then the communication has been made easy and clear, but if it is imbalanced, then you can either be too shy and quiet or too obnoxious and loud, always interrupting others.

All of the chakras work together to enhance the flow of energy within one's body, even if one chakra isn't working properly, you are still able to enhance the flow of energy using the chakras that are already in balance.

However, you go a lot of time without taking your time to work with the chakras, it may begin to even influence others around you.

For example, if you have a blocked heart chakra and you know of it but still decide to proceed with your life ignoring it and not carrying out the things that are needed to be done in order to heal and balance it, you will soon learn that you will have to deal with certain ailments that tag along with a blocked heart chakra but also that it can strongly influence the other chakras as well.

Not only that but a blocked heart chakra is known to end relationships and drift people away from each other.

Since the heart chakra is the middle major chakra, it is able to connect the chakras below and above it into one perfect flow of energy, however, if it is blocked, then the flow of energy will be far from perfect.

The heart is also responsible for sharing the flow of energy between chakras, if it is blocked it can often stop that process and block the surrounding chakras too.

Chakras have so many powers and combined, they can help us on our spiritual journey and in so many different aspects of our lives.

They are able to help us speak the truth, be truthful to one another, feel grounded in reality and on earth, feel safe and secure in life, find your purpose on earth, discover your spiritual path, enjoy some of the good things that life has to offer for you, feel the love, empathy, and compassion for not only yourself but for others too, and lastly, it can even to help you work on your psychic powers with a bonus of developing a strong connection with the universe, the physical world, the spiritual world, and your Higher-self.

There are so many things that the practice of awakening chakras can help you achieve.

Like mentioned before, high vibrations are able to attract other high vibrational things into your life.

Balancing chakras can help reach that high vibrational state that can attract anything that you wish for, anything from a lover, or a successful career full of abundance.

However, one should also be warned that opening and balancing the chakras is one thing, but having too much energy in certain chakra points can cause it to become overactive meaning there would be too much energy at that point which will cause it to become too overwhelmed.

Feelings of obsession or control can take over.

It is important that when practicing and learning to open and balance the chakras that you understand that when starting off, you are devoting yourself to this practice.

The human mind is vulnerable and can change drastically, taking the time to practice and meditate when it comes to balancing chakras can help keep the flow of energy under control.

This way, your body will get used to the natural and balanced energy and will no longer require your constant practice of everyday meditation, but rather at least once a week.

There are a lot of different ways that can help promote the balance and health of the chakras such as yoga, color therapy, crystals, affirmations, meditation, a healthy diet, and so many more things.

Even by learning to forgive others who hurt you, moving on away from your past, giving love to people, preventing yourself from speaking too much, and along with other changes in life can be used to promote a healthy flow of this energy within your body.

Opening chakras can only bring in good things into one's life unless used for selfish purposes.

There are, however, some unpleasant side effects due to your body getting used to the pure and high amount of the chakra energy but it only lasts for a couple of hours or days at most.

This practice and all of the meditations listed in this book are perfectly safe and guaranteed to work if one puts in some time, patience, and faith into the process and the universe!

Chapter 2: Benefits Of Chakra Awakening

There are a lot of benefits from awakening chakras.

By now you are very familiar with what chakras are, their importance to the body, and how a blocked chakra is able to create disease or illness within the body, but it also has the power to heal it.

Due to the imbalance in energy within the body, many illnesses and diseases are able to be born out of so much negative energy, however, pure and positive energy is known to be so much stronger than the negative one, meaning it can potentially heal and get rid of whatever illness it has created.

Not just physical illnesses but mental ones too, with the help of opening a chakra that relates to that sick region, one can form and turn their life upside down by achieving self-healing, alongside creating healthy habits and behaviors.

Many people experience a restoration of strength and energy in their physical bodies but also an increase, for example, when they go on a jog, they have the strength and energy stronger than before which helps them to run longer than their usual time.

Another benefit, which will be discussed more in another chapter, is the Kundalini awakening that can be triggered by the balance of the chakras.

The kundalini awakening is the energy of consciousness, it has been around you since before you were even born but it is located and locked deep inside of you, waiting for the right time and the right body state to re-emerge.

Just like awakening chakras, the kundalini also has countless benefits such as expanding mind power, shifting the view of reality, bringing change into one's life, making goals come true, and so much more.

The main benefit of the kundalini awakening is that it is able to balance out all of the chakras even when you haven't activated all of them.

This energy also stays within the body, never leaving, and keeping the body pure every minute of your day.

The kundalini energy can be released by itself, many times the practitioner doesn't even see it coming.

There are also many people who experience a knowledge awakening instead of an energy boost, they begin to realize that they have answers to things they don't recall reading or learning about.

This is because the information was already stored in their minds, either if they saw it on tv or overheard it from someone without paying that information any particular attention.

The mind is very independent, it can often accomplish things that even you are not aware of.

When experiencing a knowledge awakening, everything that the mind caught on begins to resurface, granting you an inner knowledge.

It is also guaranteed that learning, remembering, and taking in new information becomes so much easier as it expands the mind power.

The energies of the universe are known to be a very mysterious power!

So, why is it so important to keep these chakras cleansed and balanced?

Well, firstly it is because when the chakras are blocked, they can cause us emotional and physical ailments.

When the body is not in balance both emotionally and physically, it can start to affect the physical environment that the person is in.

When one suffers physically, it can often cause stress and unhappiness, misaligning the emotional and the physical aspects of a person.

Many times you have experienced heavy emotions directed at you or others around you within your life, this is because the chakras are imbalanced and their imbalanced emotional state is trying to release these toxic emotions, and often times it is mistakenly released on others.

When you find yourself angry or stressed, it's in human nature that everything else can enhance those feelings.

Negative feelings, especially concentrated on other people, can cause arguments, separation, hatred for one another, divorce, and overall a tense environment.

Even a lot of the physical problems that many can experience any time, such as stomach pain, headaches, and countless others, they can all be caused by an imbalance in chakras.

Know that when such physical ailments happen, they should not affect your mood drastically even though it is in human nature to be cranky when experiencing a headache.

Don't let such feelings affect your environment, if you want to release emotions, there are countless different ways that can help you such as journaling, listening to music, writing, drawing, and so many others.

Allow for your negative energy to be released and for you to be filled with calmness and peace instead.

When reacting to illnesses in a positive manner, they will also be able to disappear faster.

A lot of people are also interested in awakening their chakras because they are able to increase and promote their own psychic powers.

When awakening chakras, especially the third eye which relates to spirituality and psychic abilities, it is possible to see a vast improvement in those gifts.

Not only that but discovering other psychic gifts that you didn't even know you had until the third eye awakening.

However, you must also regard and understand that awakening psychic abilities shouldn't be your only goal.

It is simply a bonus that comes with balancing out the energies within the body.

Focus more on the spiritual journey side of the chakra awakening rather than on psychic power, this way the process won't feel forced as well as desperate, and the psychic gifts will be able to come to you more naturally.

Opening chakras can also promote Reiki healing.

Reiki is known as a healing energy that is able to heal not only yourself but other living things such as people and animals.

This pure healing energy that originated from Japan is able to not only heal the body, but the mind, spirit, and emotions too.

It is a pure spiritually guided life force energy that encourages the user to heal themselves and others with the power of Reiki symbols.

It is also able to open different chakras and balance their energy throughout the body.

Another great benefit of awakening chakras in achieving an overall balance in the body, mind, spirit, and the physical environment surrounding the practitioner.

It is like a balance between personal and working life, but instead, it balances out all of the aspects of one's life, including what goes on inside the mind.

Even just focusing on each of the chakras and devoting yourself to practice and encourage chakras qualities such as security, power, love, etc. you will be able to live up to those qualities.

They are able to manifest and turn into your reality.

Even something as simple as placing your hand on the region of that chakra while making an intention to promote security in your life, for example, which relates to the root chakra.

A balance can be achieved through the power of awareness, becoming more aware of what is happening around you and bringing your attention to become more of all the chakras can help you achieve balance.

When awakening the chakras, you are connecting to the pure energy of yourself and your Higher-self.

You are also forming a stronger connection with the spiritual world, the universe, and the divine.

The power of intuition is also awakened since all chakras are known to relate to intuition on some level.

Chakras are also able to promote motivation and inspiration to the practitioner.

Each chakra chapter will include its own separate benefits in terms of what that chakra can help you either physically or emotionally, such as improving your relationships, making your life more secure, being able to express the truth, develop the intuition ability, becoming more in touch with your emotions, and so many more.

Awakening chakras can help develop your energy flow meaning that the body's healing abilities and all the functions will be able to transform, increase, and work at a much faster rate.

The life force is known to move through the mind-body system, and this energy is also transformed into the emotional, mental, and physical expressions of your body.

A great technique in improving your weak spots when it comes to your own energy flow is by pointing out the things that you lack.

Take a look at the root chakra which is associated with support and safety, mentally one would feel confident in their life, physically healthy and stable, emotionally supported, and independent.

Examine if you have the same qualities and if you don't set a specific intention of what you want to improve when you meditate for the root chakra.

It will help you expand where you need more energy and will help you balance out the life force.

One balanced chakra can help balance out the other chakras with the help of a strong will.

Chakras are also able to help one achieve different things and goals about themselves that they wish to change or about their own environment.

Simply by setting the right intentions that relate to the right chakras can help you promote the quality that you want in yourself or accomplish a specific goal that you have in mind.

For example, if one wants to promote confidence and get rid of shyness, then meditating on the throat chakra will help with that, as well as keeping your goal in mind through that meditation.

To awaken the chakras within your body, you have to be able to enter a calm and relaxed state as well as visualize specific things unraveling before you.

Meditation is known to be a major key to many life problems, as well as the perfect guide to awakening the chakras.

When awakening your chakra, you are changing and developing yourself and your life.

Solving problems within yourself and learning to let go and leave the past where it belongs is how you are able to love yourself and others around you.

Meditation can also help you calm down and learn to control your thoughts since many of our thoughts influence the world around us, they attract different things into our lives and they shape our personalities.

Many articles and studies online concluded that meditation can help you get rid of stress, anxiety, and depression which are the main reasons and causes why certain chakras are blocked.

Not only are you calming your mind, but you are also learning to free yourself from the inner chaos of your mind.

Different chakras require a different meditation to follow which will be listed in the following chapters.

When meditating, you learn to let go of all your thoughts and negative emotions in order to open a specific chakra point but your mind also gets rid of all the toxins your brain picked up during the day and enhances what is useful.

This can help purify and balance your mind.

People always ask how much time would it take to open a chakra point and the answer is unknown.

Everyone is different and unique in their own way, no one shares the exact same thoughts as you and when it comes to opening a chakra point, your strong will is what matters the most.

It all depends on your mental and physical state but also the proper guidance for meditation.

If it doesn't work the first time then don't give up, your mind catches on the pattern so if you meditate at least once a day and practice on opening your chakra, the mind will let itself open it for you.

Repetition is the key to many things, as well as getting rid of your bad habits and healing your body.

Your mind is blind and can't tell the difference between what is real and what isn't, the proof to that is when you wake up panting and sweating from having a nightmare.

When opening chakras, you first have to get rid of any fear that is constantly clouding your vision, and in order to do that, you have to trick your mind into thinking that it is gone.

Saying affirmations always helps to change oneself and improve your way of living.

Affirmations can trick our minds into believing what we want them to believe, after all, we become whatever we constantly think of.

Many people become discouraged when they first try it and it doesn't work but what they don't understand is that this is a spiritual journey, to become aware of yourself and the universe around you.

Harnessing energy and awakening the energies of the universe can't be done overnight, the energy that it carries is bigger than the entire galaxy and the wait is worth it.

The stronger your will power to change and open your chakras, the stronger the energy to do that will be.

The meditation that will be used to help you open your chakras is called concentration meditation, which is when you focus on one point, one specific thing to help you concentrate and relax your body and mind.

Below are some tips to help you meditate that apply to all chakra points meditation but can also be used for simple and basic meditation.

Chapter 3: The Root Chakra

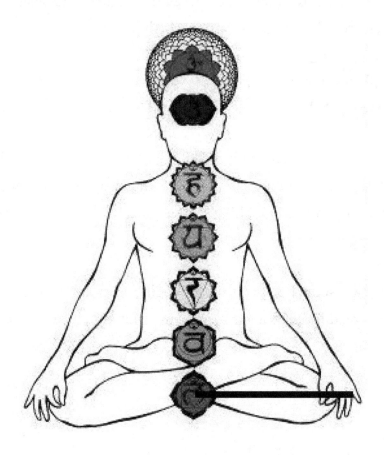

One of the very first major chakras found within the body is the root chakra.

This chakra is also known as Muladhara, 'Mula' signifying root and 'Dhara' meaning support or base.

Together, they make up the importance behind the root chakra which is to provide balance or support.

The root chakra is responsible for a sense of emotional safety and security when it comes to ones day to day activities.

It is all about survival and grounding oneself.

This chakra works by connecting your very own energy to the earth's energy through the practice of grounding oneself with the power of visualization which you will learn in this chapter.

The root chakra makes sure that you feel at ease when it comes to things such as love, goals, money, and security.

This chakra represents the color red that is associated with love, strength, security, energy, desire, and power.

It can be found in the lower abdomen, where the tailbone of the spine is located.

It makes you feel alive and brings awareness that you are being on this planet living your own life with nothing controlling you.

An imbalanced root chakra can not only damage the mind but the body too.

Physically, this chakra is associated with problems and diseases inside the spine, nerve system, the lower abdomen, kidney, hemorrhoids, and sleep disorders.

One may also suffer from pain, bladder issues, digestion problems, ovarian cysts, and lower back pains.

When emotionally imbalanced, one will live their life worrying about almost anything every single day.

Negative feelings like anxiety, insecurity, impatience, and stress will resurface causing other mental illnesses such as depression.

Since the flow of energy is blocked, that energy will not properly reach the legs causing one to always feel exhausted after walking.

When your root chakra is balanced, you will live a life free of worries, situations that refer to your survival requirements won't stress you, and you will be able to react to different circumstances with a calm mindset.

The trust is found within yourself, you believe that you can get through any obstacles without it interfering with your mental health.

Physically, when this chakra is balanced, the body is healthy and energized.

There are no difficulties relating to the lower abdomen.

Emotionally, this chakra deals with anxiety and stress so when it is in balance, those feelings simply fade away.

With a positive mindset, no negative thoughts, and the root chakra can help achieve a mental balance as well as balancing other chakras such as the sacral and the heart by getting rid of negative emotions.

The reaction to obstacles and problems will improve without a panic state of mind state.

Chakras can also be either overactive or underactive, meaning that its either too open which can affect one not in a good way or it's not open enough.

When the root chakra is overactive, the root chakra can also create 'threats' inside your mind, making you believe in it when in reality there is nothing that can harm you.

These threats will cause paranoia, leading to jittery and anxious.

You will also find yourself getting aggressive, annoyed, and angry all the time.

The slightest provocation will tick you off. This type of person always tries to control others for their greedy deeds.

They often resist higher authority, change, and are known to obsess over feeling secure.

When the root chakra is underactive, then it means that one has taken care of the survival needs but not in a healthy manner.

It is not 'open enough' meaning that one still feels disconnected or insecure when it comes to the outside world.

They easily feel nervous, anxious, afraid, and find it hard to finish daily tasks on time.

In order to balance this chakra, one must also consider changing daily habits to help assist in the opening of this chakra.

A change in diet can strongly influence the mind, body, and root chakra.

A healthy and well-balanced diet can help achieve mental clarity, provide health for the body, and even help balance the root chakra.

Try to consume healthy foods and drink a lot of water, it is not only beneficial for the root chakra but can even help to prevent any unwanted diseases within the body.

Especially eating red foods such as tomatoes, strawberries, red peppers, and many others can help assist in the opening of the root chakra.

Exercising like jogging, hiking, or yoga can help the body's health and the root chakra.

An open root chakra will make you feel grounded and more confident in yourself.

Meditation is known to be one of the best ways to awaken and open the root chakra, but before beginning with this meditation, one should ground themselves first.

Grounding can help the person connect to the earth more which is what this chakra is all about.

A perfect way to ground oneself is by walking barefooted in nature, the beach, or the forest.

Walking barefooted at home can also help.

Another popular way is to use the power of visualization by imagining yourself as an energy tree by extending your arms upwards.

Visualize roots below you, sinking deeper into the ground, and the branches above you, extending from your hands.

This is a brief visualization exercise and it can help ground you.

It shouldn't take longer than two to three minutes, it can also help calm the mind before you get into the meditation state.

Meditation For The Root Chakra

Begin by getting comfortable in the meditation sacred place of your choosing.

This time, instead of laying down, you will be sitting with your legs crossed.

Make sure that your spine and shoulders are straight and tall which will be more effective when healing the lower abdomen and the root chakra.

Allow for your hands to rest on your knees, with the palms facing up.

Form your hands into the mudra hand position by forming a circle using your thumb and your index finger, it can also be interpreted as an okay hand gesture.

Begin to breathe deeply, inhale and hold the breath for three seconds before exhaling it and dragging it out for another three seconds.

Make sure that when you are breathing in and out that you use your chest, rather than breathing in through your stomach.

When you are using the chest, the spine extends and moves along with the breathing, this will enable the relaxation of the body even when you are sitting up.

Take a few minutes to simply relax your muscles and the body as you breathe in.

Bring your attention to your breathing as you inhale and exhale to help calm the mind.

Try your best to not listen to your thoughts and the mental clutter that is going on inside your head.

Instead, bring your focus to yourself as a being in this big universe.

Don't think about anything else that you have to do or things that might be bothering, instead focus on breathing through your chest, making the lungs expand as you breathe in.

Take some time to bring your attention to different parts of your body, relaxing them in the process.

Think of your face muscles, relaxing as they tingle with your life force energy that you always have within you.

Then bring your attention to your arms, legs, belly, and other parts of your body that you might feel some tension in.

Allow yourself to feel the different tingling sensations all throughout as you let your body go numb and relax.

Gradually bring your attention back to your breathing, notice how your chest rises and falls every time you inhale or exhale.

Allow your eyes to lightly close, as if you are slowly falling into a deep slumber.

Create a breathing pattern, it is often related to how you would breathe normally.

Slow down your breathing by holding it in and extending it one or two seconds longer when you breathe out.

When you take a deep breath in, notice how the air travels down into your lower belly and then back up through your nose as you exhale.

Deeply breathe in and out a few times before bringing your awareness to the location of the root chakra, the base of your spine where your tailbone is.

Focus on your breathing and don't let your mind slip away as you allow for your energy to awaken.

Begin to resurface the energy within you by visualizing your body glowing white, the white that represents your pure energy that is deeply in connection with your soul.

The white begins to surround your body, circulating and connecting with your aura.

Rest in that sensation for another minute or two before concentrating and directing that energy into the palms of your hands.

Center the flow of energy into your palms, by imagining it all flowing to your hands as it travels from different parts of your body, like arms and legs.

Let yourself feel any tingling sensations or warmth.

Allow it to rest there, forming a white ball of light in each of your hands.

Lift your hands up and place them down on your lower abdomen.

Imagine the light and energy that you have gathered begin to change color, from a pure white into a red while allowing it to enter through the lower abdomen and into the root chakra.

Red is associated with the root chakra and using this color can help not only open the chakra but also direct the energy into that specific area.

Visualize that red light enters your chakra point and the healing energy that is being sent with it.

Inhale and contract the muscles between the pubic bone and the tailbone as the light enters, engaging the Mula Bandha that can help to further activate your energy and release the root chakra energy.

You are drawing the perineum towards the root chakra.

Bring your attention to how the Mula Bandha feels as you breathe flows in and your muscles contract.

Hold your breath for one to two seconds before releasing the Mula Bandha and relaxing your muscles.

Repeat again by tightening and contracting the muscles once again, feel how your spine becomes taller, pulling you up while pushing your legs and feet down.

Let go after one or two seconds and let your muscles relax again.

Repeat for at least two to three minutes or however long you seem it fit.

As you release the contract, the root chakra energy increases.

Visualize the energy intercepting with that of the root chakra, connecting and expanding further.

Allow for your body to fall into a state of relaxation, you might find it even more relaxing than when you started your meditation.

Let that energy simply travel around the lower abdomen.

You might feel some tingling sensations or warmth down your spine or throughout your body, this indicates that your chakra is being opened and the body is experiencing high energies.

Let that red light circulate in the lower abdomen, cleansing out all of the negative energy within that area.

Then, continue the healing process by imagining that red light traveling down your crossed legs as you are sitting up, connecting with the muscles and relaxing any tensions that you might have.

Allow for it to travel back up into the lower abdomen, resting there and releasing all the tensions before allowing it to travel back down again.

This time, as it makes its way all the way down to the souls of your feet, imagine that energy leaving your body through the bottom of where you are located.

If you are sitting on a bed, or on the floor, imagine that energy reaching out into the ground, as if you are a tree and the red energy is your roots.

Let it rest in that sensation, grounding you and connecting with the energy from the earth's element.

Feel the earth's energy connect with your own, intercepting and becoming one before allowing your red root energies to return back to your through the souls of your feet.

Let that magnified energy to travel back up to your lower abdomen, letting it rest there as you take notice of any tensions within your lower abdomen or your legs.

If you feel any tensions or tingling, then allow for that energy to go there.

Let the energy rest in that area while you imagine healing and banishment of any tensions or negativity.

If there are any other tensions within the root chakra area, then allow for the energy to travel there.

The glow is expanding, making you feel warm and relaxed.

Feel the root chakra, feel any sensations, warmth, or tingling in the tailbone area.

Gently rest in the sensations for a few minutes as you breathe in deeply.

Once you feel relaxed and good about your healing, return the energy to the lower abdomen.

Bring your attention back to your breathing as you bring your awareness back into your body.

Take a minute to simply breathe and stay present at this moment.

Allow for your eyes to slowly open, adjusting them to the light and the physical world around you.

Consider laying down somewhere or continue sitting up if you wish, but take some time to reflect and think back to your meditation before proceeding with your day.

When you are done, thank the universe for guiding you and for helping you heal yourself.

Take some time to relax after the healing process, don't push yourself to do anything.

Stay at home, relax, take a hot bath, and let your body heal itself while the energy within your body is still present.

Chapter 4: The Sacral Chakra

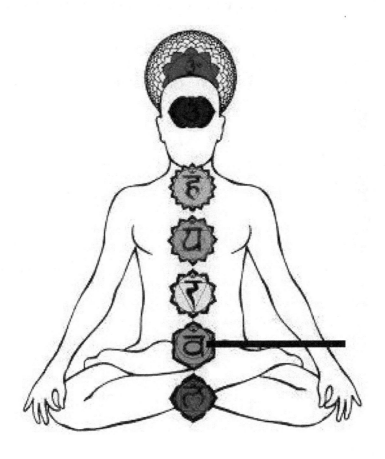

The second major chakra is the sacral chakra.

It is also known as Svadhishana which signifies 'the place of the self'.

In context, this chakra is all about making you feel like you belong in this world.

It gives you the feelings and emotions that make you enjoy your life, as well as living with creative energy that makes up your persona.

This chakra provides the feeling of satisfaction and survival which comes from the root chakra.

The sacral chakra is responsible for one's inner feelings that make up the happiness, it is also responsible for all of the emotional aspect of a person.

It represents connection, intimacy, pleasure, and sensuality.

The sacral chakra is associated with the color orange which represents creativity, joy, success, and self-respect.

The location of this chakra is below the belly button in the lower abdomen region which mostly affects that specific region within the body.

When imbalanced, a person will experience extreme difficulties when it comes to both the mind and body.

Physically, one will suffer from problems within the reproductive system, kidney infections, urinary problems, prostate problems, constipation, hormonal imbalance, gynecological problems, abnormal menstruation in females, and problems within the sexual organs.

This chakra is also the cause of one's negative addictions and emotions.

In order to be healthy, one must first realize that negative actions have negative consequences.

Ask yourself if what you are doing is good for your health.

Change starts from within the mind by drawing the energy away from what you are addicted to.

Emotionally, one will suffer from negative feelings, weakness, insecurity, and fear, which will then affect the root chakra and its feelings of security.

One will also find themselves to be enjoying things that shouldn't be the main cause of one's happiness.

New addictions will resurface as well as lack of motivation, restlessness, emotional confusion, and feelings of unimportance.

However, when this chakra is balanced, it lets one stay and live in the moment, experiencing all the wonderful feelings that come with it.

The sacral chakra let's one understand the things that life offers and that everything happens for a reason.

Physically, the lower abandonment region such as the reproductive organs, bladder, and stomach suffer no physical pain.

The energy within the body is also well balanced, meaning one will never feel tired or exhausted.

Emotionally, one will be able to express themselves easily since this chakra is linked to the feelings and emotions of the mind.

The emotional state will be well-balanced meaning that when situations will get heated, you will not overreact which is known to often cause more stress.

When this chakra is overactive, the sacral may be experiencing too much energy causes an imbalance to the sacral chakra region.

When it happens, the overall well-being of a person is affected.

One will experience conflict, drama, and unhealthy relationships as well as constant overwhelming feelings.

The emotions will be expressed more deeply, they will also be heightened.

Moodswings, a strong dependence on others, attachment, aggression, anxiety, and emotional imbalance are common side effects of an overactive sacral chakra.

When the sacral chakra is underactive, then one is most likely experiencing a disturbance in the flow of energy.

You will begin to suffer from losing control, feelings of uncertainty, and inability to cope with changes and obstacles in your life.

It often affects the environment and personal relationships with friends, family, and lovers.

You will feel detached from your emotions causing drastic changes for yourself and others.

Changing your diet, adding yoga, and meditation into your daily routine can only help if you let it.

Keeping an open mindset can also be of use to make sure that all the little things that one does will help in healing the sacral chakra.

One must first welcome change into their lives in order to be healed completely.

The sacral chakra is often associated with water meaning that drinking plenty of water and/or herbal teas especially fruity ones can help heal and balance this chakra point.

Eating orange foods such as oranges, melons, coconuts, and other sweet fruits can be beneficial in aiding to balance this chakra.

Foods that are orange in color can also be of help.

Specific practices such as yoga and particular yoga pose that involve opening the hips like open-angle pose, bound angle pose, and upavistha konasana are not only good for the body but can help open the sacral chakra.

Meditation For The Sacral Chakra

Find a comfortable position while you are laying down preferably in the area that can become your meditational sacred place.

When you lay down, make sure to place a pillow under your head so you will not fall asleep, and another pillow, rolled-up preferably, under your knees to support your legs.

Your body will notice that it is not your usual sleeping position which will make you stay awake.

Turn off your phone and lock your doors to ensure that you will not get distracted.

When you lay down, strengthen your body, facing up and begin by breathing deeply. Keep your hands on your sides, with the palms facing upwards.

Start off by focusing your attention on the way your body moves as you inhale or exhale.

Relax your arms, legs, belly, and other parts of your body where you feel most tension in.

Gradually let your eyes close themselves, slowly and not forcefully.

Make sure to maintain balanced breathing, smooth, deep and slow.

Slowly begin to close your eyes gently, not forcefully.

Allow for your body to feel as if it's entering the deepest state of relaxation while the mind and the soul are wide awake.

Continue to breathe in and out, focusing on the way your chest rises and falls with every breath you take in.

If you find your mind wandering around, simply bring it back to your body and your attention to your breathing.

Take a couple of minutes to silence your mind, getting rid of any mental clutter and bringing the mind to a state of relaxation and meditation.

Once you relax your body, bring your awareness to how your stomach and organs expand as you breath in and out.

Feel any sensations or tingling inside where your sacral chakra is located at the lower abdomen, in your pelvic region.

Breathe slowly and deeply and try to notice any changes in the area of your focus.

Can you feel your pelvic organs pulsating or tingling as you breathe?

Continue to breathe deeply, relaxing your body in the process and observing your lower abdomen.

Bring your attention to the way you breathe in, as your organs are expanding and changing their shape when you inhale or exhale.

Imagine your kidneys, and other organs moving in your body slightly as if swaying from side to side.

Begin to call out to the universe and ask to resurface the life force energy from within you.

Ask for guidance and support while setting your intention to achieve constant healing within the sacral area, the gut, and the stomach.

Allow for that energy to resurface while imagining yourself glowing white color.

Feel the flow of energy throughout your body, resurfacing, recharging the body, and getting rid of any impurities.

Thank the energy within you as it constantly moves and tries its best to heal you physically, emotionally, and spiritually.

Form a Gassho with your hands and place them in front of you where your heart is.

Focus on centering the energy into your hands as you ask for guidance and healing from the Universe.

Once you've gathered energy white and pure energy within your hands, proceed by pressing them down onto your sacrum, the lower abdomen stomach area, that is a couple of inches below the belly button.

This is where the Sacral chakra resigns.

Allow that energy to hover in the sacral chakra, opening it and freeing its own energy.

Place your hands on the lower abdomen, skin to skin, and feel any sensations or movements through your hands.

Visualize the warmth radiating from both sides of the skin, picture an orange glow lighting up and warming up your hands.

You will start to feel tingling and movements in your lower abdomen.

Let it move all throughout your stomach and gut area, visualize receiving healing, improving your digestion, or even increasing your intuition, the gut feeling.

Lift your hands up and place them on your mind.

Visualize sending the healing energy into the mind, imagine opening it and balancing your emotions.

Think of all the negative energy simply letting go and moving on.

Replace those negative feelings that are letting themselves leave your body with those of happiness by thinking back to your happiest memories or about things that make you happy.

This will let the body experience its 'true' and happy state.

Imagine the light evolving and glowing brighter and brighter, radiating from your hands with the feeling of warmth and tingling sensations around that area whether you have physical contact with the skin or are simply allowing your hands to hover above.

Remove your hands and place them back on your lower stomach, the region that connects to feelings of enjoyment of living and happiness.

Allow for yourself to enjoy and live in this moment, notice the butterflies and the joyous feelings they give out in your stomach.

Each time you deeply inhale, bring that orange glow a tiny bit brighter and bigger.

Feel the creative and inspirational energy run through your veins.

Lay in that feeling for a few minutes before gently opening your eyes.

Breathe in the air around you and look around as you still feel that strong and bright energy.

Clear this area for about two to three minutes before placing one of your hands on your back, with the palms facing downwards.

Proceed to visualize further healing and opening of this chakra.

Allow for the energy to travel all around, to any tensions within the area and banishing any impurities.

Visualize cleansing and purifying the mind by healing and opening the Sacral chakra.

Hold your hands there for two to three minutes at most, resting your mind as you breathe in deeply and slowly.

Consider taking some time to gently massage the area to promote a healthy flow of energy, relaxation, and freedom of any tension.

If you choose to massage the area then make sure you do it clockwise for women and anticlockwise for men, or whichever way feels right to you.

Gently press three fingers, the index finger, the middle finger, and the ring finger against your exposes stomach.

Begin by gently applying pressure before massaging it in a circular way.

Proceed by breathing in deeply, holding in the breath for three seconds before letting go as you massage it.

Continue to visualize the orange healing energy swimming within the area that you touch, healing it in the process.

Slowly bring your attention back to your breathing, allowing for the energy to evenly spread back throughout your body while cleansing it and removing any impurities.

Rest for a minute before gently opening your eyes.

Allow yourself to lay in the feeling of being aware of your surroundings for a couple of minutes while reminding yourself of your pure intentions of healing yourself while cleansing the body with the energy.

Reflect on your meditation.

Did you receive any sensations or visions?

Often times during meditations especially with healing, the universe might speak through visions to hint something else that might be needed for healing, either physical or mental.

Breathe in the air around you and look around as you might be filled with strong and bright energy.

This new found energy might overwhelm you with a strong urge to create, so allow it to guide you in releasing the energy through creating some with inspiration.

Chapter 5: The Solar Plexus Chakra

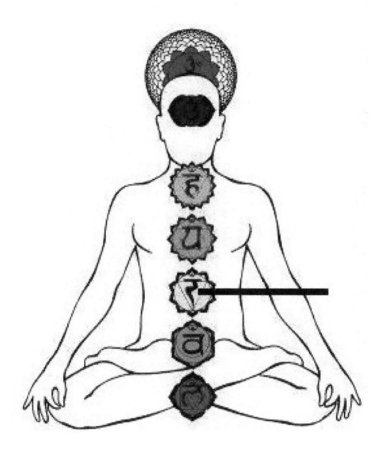

The third chakra point is the solar plexus, it is also referred to as Manipura which means 'lustrous gem' and 'resplendent gem'.

Since the chakra is located in the upper abdomen, just a couple of inches above your belly button, it is known as chakra of intuition, or 'gut feeling' due to its location.

This chakra is the representation of one's willpower and the strong desire to achieve success.

It is also associated with wisdom, confidence, and the perception of who you are as a person.

The solar plexus is the origin of one's self-discipline and self-esteem that makes up a person as a whole.

It turns thoughts and goals into actions through willpower.

This chakra is associated with the color yellow which means energetic, cheerful, happiness, intellect, and encouragement.

When the solar plexus is imbalanced, the energy is either directed too much on the body or mind.

Physically, the solar plexus is responsible for the problems found within the muscular system, the cellular respiration, the nervous system, digestive system, blood sugar problems, hypertension, and gallbladder.

When this chakra is imbalanced emotionally, one will always suffer from migraines, changes in attitude, mood imbalance, and lack of motivation.

You will also begin to feel powerless in situations within your life, like losing control of everything that happens around you.

This will cause you to always be angry or lashing out to surrounding people, applying negative energy to the environment and influencing other people negatively.

Life will become a hassle rather than being filled with joy and living it to the fullest.

When balanced, one feels as if they have the power to accomplish any of their goals, this strong feeling is able to turn the thoughts into actions.

The balanced solar plexus chakra makes you feel full of energy, lively and gives you the ability to accomplish challenges.

You are confident in yourself and your power to follow through the difficulties that life throws at you while making sure that the mind stays in a calm, cheerful, and confident state.

Physically, the body is healthy and fit due to the fact that the solar plexus has all the control over the cellular respiration system within the body.

This makes sure that the body is in great condition and health.

The flow of energy throughout the body is balanced and strong, also aiding in the healing process of the body.

Emotionally, this chakra can ease the worries of the mind as well as releasing it and other negative feelings, maintaining the mind clear, healthy and well-balanced along with the body.

A balance in the solar plexus promotes strength, motivation, courage, and happiness in the body, mind, and soul, thus enabling this chakra to balance out the other major chakras.

When the solar plexus is underactive, it will disturb the flow of energy within the body.

You may start to experience a lack of control as well as a loss of purpose in life.

This often leads to a lot of emotional problems, self-destructive behavior, and self-doubt.

Underactive solar plexus makes one feel helpless, indecisive, grants a low-esteem, and a lack of confidence.

When the solar plexus is overactive, it means that the solar plexus has way too much energy in the region compared to other chakras.

You will experience issues in controlling people, yourself, and your environment.

Having control over your own life is good as long as it is not going overboard which an overactive solar plexus does.

When it is overactive, you will feel overwhelmed in energy that can overstimulate the system and tire the body out.

One will also become stubborn, aggressive, judgmental, and overcritical.

This chakra is best to be opened with meditation but adding certain changes in diet can also help greatly.

Eating yellow-based foods such as grains, yellow peppers, bananas, and corn, as well as other complex carbohydrate foods that are able to give you plenty of energy can help in the opening of the solar plexus.

However, you must avoid too many sugary foods seeing as the glucose is not natural.

Make sure to drink plenty of chamomile tea which is known to help clear the blockage of this chakra.

Decorating one's house with yellow flowers or wearing yellow clothing can help stimulate the solar plexus visually.

Meditation For The Solar Plexus Chakra

Begin with a light stretch, too relax the muscles for your meditation.

Stand up, and lift your hands up into the air as if you are reaching up to touch the sky.

Reach as far as you can while you take a deep breath in, holding the position and your breath for two seconds.

As you exhale, drop your hands to your sides, pulling the breath for another two seconds.

Lift your hands up again as you breathe in and drop them to your sides as you exhale.

Repeat at least three times before proceeding with the meditation.

Sit up in a comfortable position on the floor or on a chair in the room of your sacral chakra meditation healing practice.

Cross your legs, as you extend your spine nice and straight.

Lift your head up, as if you are balancing a book right on top.

Place your hands on your knees with the palms facing upwards.

Get rid of any distraction, by closing the windows, turning off your phone, and locking the doors.

Start off your meditation by breathing slowly and deeply while staring off into space.

Take as long as you need to relax your body, muscles, and adjust your mind from wandering around and gently allow for your eyes to slowly close.

Further bring your body to relaxation by focusing on and relaxing different parts of your body such as legs, stomach, chest, arms, shoulders, neck and head, as you move your focus along your body from top to bottom.

Take a couple of seconds to hold the image of yourself sitting up, while you are relaxing your body.

You can also direct your focus to how your chest and body rise taller as you breathe in or falls shorter as you breathe out.

Hold your attention on your breathing to ensure that your mind won't slip away.

By bringing your focus somewhere else except your mind, you are able to clear your thoughts from any worries of troubles.

Now that your body is close to its relaxed state and so is your mind, change the way you breathe to fit the opening of the solar plexus area.

Since the location of the chakra is on the lower part of your ribs, you will be using your chest to breath.

Inhale the air and expand your lungs, hold the breath for at least four seconds before exhaling through your mouth.

Visualize releasing any negativity through your exhale as your spine expands higher every time you breathe.

Focus on the way your chest rises and falls and don't let your mind wander away.

If it does, then gently bring your attention back to your attention to the movement of the spine.

Just like any other healing treatments, call on the Universe and ask to heal your solar plexus chakra.

Visualize channeling your energy and centering it on the palm of your hands.

Allow for the energy to resurface your body, as a white pure life force healing energy.

Let it hover all throughout your body for a minute, energizing it and gathering its strength.

Place your hands on the area above your belly button but below your heart.

You will be touching the lower part of your ribs.

You should place your hands next to each other and not overlapping each other.

Concentrate on making the energy flow through your hands and to the solar plexus.

Visualize it healing the chakra, clearing it of any blockage and releasing the negative emotions or negative tensions that could possibly affect the physical health of the body, imagine anything negative leaving through your mouth as you exhale.

When you are sitting down, start to connect and feel the coldness or warmth of the floor, the bed, or the ground beneath you.

Visualize the energy from the ground traveling up through your body, through your toes.

Imagine sucking in that energy that belongs to the earth.

Focus on this energy as it's moving up towards the location of the solar plexus which is in between your belly button and the bottom of your rib cage, also known as the upper abdomen.

With your hands still on the upper abdomen, imagine yellow glow forming and expanding in that area as all the energy begin connecting, rotating clockwise and getting larger every time you take a breath in.

Feel the warmth and sensation that the yellow light is providing and how it makes you feel emotional.

Keep your hands on that area for at least two to three minutes before moving on and placing your hands on the top of your knees, forming a mudra by touching both the thumb and the index finger together.

If you'd like, you can keep cleansing the area for longer than three minutes, however long you feel is necessary for your upper abdomen to heal.

Begin to imagine that you are sitting on top of a grassy hill, sitting right below the sun that is shinning right back down on you.

Your eyes are closed as your own sacral chakra begins to glow and react with the sun.

The energy tingling within your upper abdomen, experiencing healing and cleansing.

Focus your attention on the part of your body that you imagine is the warmest from the sun, such as the top of your head.

Yellow stimulates the feelings of joy and it also represents the solar plexus.

Feel and appreciate the warmth that you are receiving and accept the tingling sensations that are spreading through your body.

Then start to bring your attention inwards, notice how the ground beneath you feels like, is it cold or warm?

Can you feel any tingling or pulses through it?

What about the space above your head?

Does it feel like a whole universe is right above you just by feeling a little pressure on your head?

Freely lift your arms up towards the sky as you inhale and feel the astral world above you.

Picture a bright yellow flame at the tip of your fingers, feel as it connects through your hands and travels down to your upper abandonment where the solar plexus is located.

Breath out and lower your arms down to the ground.

Place your hands on the ground and feel the earth beneath you and the perfect balance of life and energy around you.

Inhale once more, raising your hands up towards the sky as if connecting your energy with the one with the sun.

Let the yellow glow travel down to you upper abandonment, clearing and opening that chakra point.

Notice what you are feeling during this moment, are you feel calm, balanced and happy?

Repeat the hand motions for a few minutes or however long you wish.

Place your hands back down on your knees, forming the mudra. Use the mantra 'ram' by saying it out loud physically.

This specific mantra vibrates the body and helps the negative energies flow out of the chakra and out of the body while leaving only positive and pure healing forces.

Mantras are just words that are said during meditations but it can also be used in practices to ensure that the body is cleared effectively.

Place one of your hands on your back, with the palm facing outwards while you repeat the same process of visualizing the yellow energy healing moving and releasing any tensions in the upper abdomen.

Take a minute to rest in the healing sensations.

To finish, place your hands back to the ground.

Breath in deeply with an open mind for a minute while bringing your awareness back to the physical world.

Imagine the room that you are in to help get back to your consciousness and the body.

Make an intention to express utmost gratitude to the Universe for guidance, your energy for healing you, and opening your solar plexus chakra.

Take another minute to simply breathe in deeply, in through your nose and out through your mouth.

Open your eyes slowly but do not move your body.

Look around you, take in the details of your room, stay in the moment for a few minutes while reflecting on the healing that you just achieved.

Chapter 6: The Heart Chakra

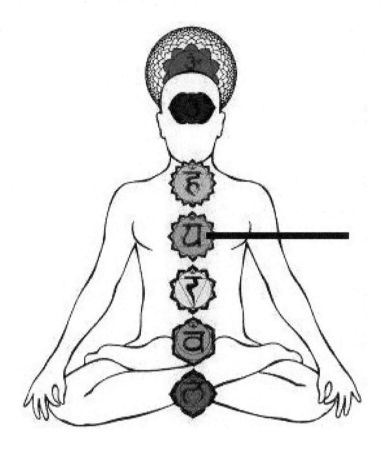

The fourth major chakra point is the heart chakra, also known as Anahata chakra that means 'unhurt'.

The context of the meaning connected to the heart chakra, when it is healthy and in balance, the heart and mind are not hurt.

The heart chakra connects to the mind, it is also the source of the deepest emotions such as unconditional love, compassion, passion, and joy.

The feelings of the heart are able to be expressed through the throat chakra and the mind, those deep feelings that are sometimes very hard to express verbally come from the heart.

Since the heart is the middle chakra, it connects the chakras below it and to the chakras above it.

The heart chakra is associated with the color green which represents prosperity, wealth in any aspect of one's life, health, and abundance.

This chakra can help heal both mental and physical issues.

The location of the heart chakra is right in the middle of the chest area.

When imbalanced, the heart experiences many negative emotions and negative energy in the body, mind, and the physical environment due to the fact that low vibrations attract other low vibration.

Negative thoughts and emotions can also cause the proper function of the body to fail.

Physically, the heart chakra is responsible for the problems found in the immune system, the circulatory system, respiratory system, muscle, and diaphragm.

Illnesses such as breast cancer, lung diseases, heart disease, allergies, asthma, high blood pressure, and other health problems revolving the heart chakra region.

Emotionally, this chakra deals with very deep emotions such as grief, anxiety, jealousy, hatred, loneliness, fear, and isolation, especially when the heart chakra is imbalanced.

You will always feel like you are stuck in the past or constantly thinking about the future, unable to focus on the present and what is really important at this time.

Negative feelings can cloud one's judgment, making one feel like they must always protect themselves when in fact there is no danger.

Negative emotions can also strongly impact the physical environment, causing separation, abandonment, and emotional abuse.

When in balance, you feel comfortable and healthy both physically, mentally, and spiritually.

When it is in balance, the body and mind are also at an equal with no worries, which satisfies one spiritually.

You are able to find forgiveness in your heart to those who hurt you in the past, which is also a great way to move on from that situation that left a mark on your heart.

Being stuck in the past doesn't help one focus on the present which is all life is about, enjoying and living in the moment.

The heart chakra grants compassion, peace, comfort, and gratitude for every little thing you have.

Physically, the heart is located within the heart chakra.

The heart is healthy, as well as the surrounding areas such as breasts, lungs, and ribs when the heart chakra is in balance.

It is also responsible for keeping us alive by promoting the beat of the heart and the blood circulation.

Emotionally, the heart chakra is known to be quite vulnerable but when it is in balance, one is able to experience the true meaning of happiness and what it is like to live their life filled with love and acceptance.

The mind is known to be in a very calm, confident, loving, and cheerful state.

However, that can also be the heart chakras undoing, being too cheerful and loving can sometimes backfire if it is given to the wrong people.

The underactive heart chakra revolves around the unhealthy distribution of the flow of energy within the body.

You will begin to experience an inability to forgive, forget, and move on with your life which will cause you to always be stuck in the past.

It can also prevent you from creating new relationships and opening your heart to more people.

This detaches you from the outside love as well as leaving you feeling withdrawn, isolated, critical of yourself and others.

The overactive heart chakra is distributing way too much energy, meaning that one can be giving away too much love and not leaving any for themselves.

This can leave you feeling emotionally drained and can affect your physical health.

An overactive heart chakra can lead you to feel a lack of discernment, especially in relationships as well as leave you feeling like you overexert yourself in terms of your personal life, this can make your relationships become toxic.

You will also find yourself feeling under control of your emotions and create a dependence on the personal relationships that you have with people rather than relying on yourself to be happy.

The overactive heart chakra can also cause a loss in personal boundaries, loss of identity, neglect, and always saying yes, even to things that can bring you pain.

Many times the main problems of having a blocked heart chakra revolve around a question, 'are you giving the same amount of love to yourself that you give to others' or 'are you putting yourself and your needs before anyone else'.

Many of those who have a blocked heart chakra either put other people before themselves or block their own heart from receiving love.

In order to open the heart chakra, one has to practice self-love and putting themselves before anyone else.

Your feelings and your own happiness are what matters most in the end.

Take some time to relax and gather your thoughts, follow the path which makes you the happiest self rather than pleasing and doing what other people want you to do.

Eating plenty of nutritious foods, especially those that are of green color, can help encourage the healing of the heart chakra.

Performing small acts of kindness such as smiling at a stranger or complimenting them can not only give out love but receive in the process.

No matter how much love one gives out, it will always find its way back to them in different shapes or sizes.

Opening your heart chakra will make you feel hopeful for the future, your relationships will strengthen with the people that you love and you will be able to attract more people into your life so place the stone above your heart or wear it as a necklace.

Meditation For The Heart Chakra

The key to healing the heart and chest area is through music.

Begin by picking a soft melody with gentle beats and sounds, no lyrics so you won't be able to sing along in your head.

It is scientifically proven that the right music can make you feel happier so make sure you find something that you feel a certain connection to.

Turn it on by a few bars that are soft enough to hear but not that loud, for example, 1/4 of the music bars.

Make sure that the melody is longer than ten minutes or on repeat.

Begin by laying down and relaxing comfortably.

Place a pillow under your head, and another under your knees for utmost comfort.

Leave your hands laying next to your body with the palms facing up.

Take a minute to focus and clear your mind by breathing in deeply.

Breathe in from your nose, hold the breath for two seconds and exhale through your mouth.

Continue this easy and simple breathing technique for a minute.

Inhale through the nose, and exhale through the mouth while setting a mental intention to relax your body as much as you can.

Proceed by gently closing your eyes and giving all of your attention to your chest area.

Use your lungs when you are breathing, instead of your stomach.

This means that when you breathe in, allow for your lungs to expand, moving around, filling up with oxygen.

Make sure that all of your attention is centered on your chest and the way it rises and falls or the way your body stretches upwards as you breathe in or shrinks as you breathe out.

Imagine that with every breath you take, you clear out the negativity within the chest, releasing it through the mouth, and allowing for yourself to let go of any tensions or impurities.

As you allow for your body to relax further and as you become more familiar with the deep breathing rhythm of your body, begin to listen carefully to the different tunes that you hear and try to focus on a specific one that stands out to you.

For example, if it's the sound of the bells you hear, then bring your focus there.

Try to push away any thoughts that might be emerging to the back of your head and relax while listening to that soft and quiet sound.

Take a moment to appreciate the music that you are hearing.

Observe how that melody makes you feel emotionally, are you feeling happiness and love in your heart, if so then continue by visualizing your heart fluttering as if it is opening up to love.

Think of flower petals emerging through your heart, floating around you ready to travel to your loved ones.

Keep in touch with your own emotion of love and connect it to the flower petals.

Think of a person close to you, a friend, a lover, or a family member, think of sending them those pink or green glowing petals filled with your love and empathy.

Wish them happiness and abundance through their life.

Picture those petals flowing to wherever they are now and connecting with their hearts.

Do this with two or three other people that you hold close to your heart.

Feel the warmth and tingling as more petals leave your heart and travel to your loved ones.

Let the energy gathered within your heart be released through your body, spread love throughout it and feel it within you.

Let the energy run freely up and down your spine through all the chakras, uniting them and growing your spiritual growth.

Proceed by making an intention to resurface the energy and asking the universe for guidance in this practice.

Focus on the white auric field surrounding your body, making you feel safe and comfortable.

You will begin to feel tingling sensations and warmth in different parts of your body.

Let the healing energy take its time resurfacing within your body and allow for it to center exactly where the heart is.

As you preformed the petal release exercise, the heart became more pure and positive, allowing for the energy to access it easier.

Place an intention to receive protection from anything negative in your life, negative events, negative emotions, and negative people.

This will help you feel safer and at ease from negativity.

Place another intention of receiving self-healing energy targeting the specific part of your body, the chest.

Allow for that energy to move from the heart to the shoulders and down to the palms of your hands, all connecting with one another.

Channel your energy and concentrate on centering it on your hands.

Allow the flow of white energy to resurface in your palms and glow a white and pure color.

Take a minute to just let all of the energy to catch up and gather in that area, healing the hands along the way.

Lift both of your hands and place them on your heart, one over the other.

Allow the energy to sink into your heart chakra and visualize the white-colored light changing into a bright green which is associated with the heart chakra.

Focus on feeling the beat of your heart against your hands, feel the pulsing vibrations underneath.

Rest in the moment as that green light sink in deeper into your chest.

Allow the energy to circulate and explore the chest area, going exactly where tensions are present.

Feel the tingling sensations throughout your body, smell the air around you as you take in deep breaths, hear the soft melody echoing in the room or against your ears, taste the freedom and the love life gives you and finally, although your eyes are closed, notice the glowing green light emerging through your heart.

Visualize the color glowing brighter and brighter as it opens your heart chakra to all the love and happiness that you deserve.

Think of the people who you care deeply for, imagine sending them your love and blessing to ensure that they are safe and happy with their life.

Think of different times when love was expressed and given to you, even the small things that made you happy still count!

Open yourself to healing within your heart.

Use the mantra 'yam' to help you open this chakra further.

Spend some time to opening your chakra, don't rush through the process but let your body heal its heart, either physically or emotionally.

Finish up by deeply breathing in and out through your mouth for a few minutes, just focusing on the music and the emotional feelings you receive from it.

The point of this meditation is to make you feel love to live, love for others around you, especially for yourself, and healing your chest area with positive and pure energy.

When you think you have finished, take some time for the energy to settle in within your body for a minute or two.

Allow for your eyes to slowly open, adjusting them to the light and the physical world around you.

Make sure to reflect on the meditation that you have just performed and the healing that you have received.

Proceed by doing something that makes you happy or something that you love.

Take some time to relax after the healing process, don't push yourself to do anything.

Stay at home, relax, take a hot bath, and let your body heal itself while the energy within your body is still present.

Chapter 7: The Throat Chakra

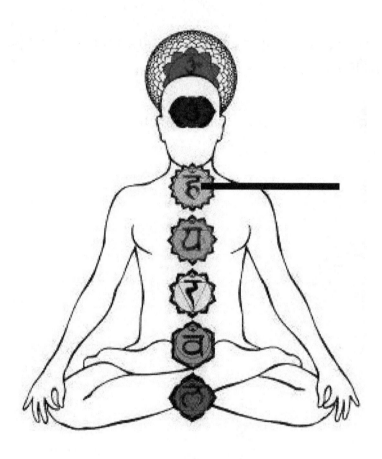

The fifth major chakra is the throat chakra that is also called Vishuddha.

Vishuddha means purification or very pure, and it signifies one having a pure mindset.

This connects to the throat chakra because, in order to have a pure mind, one must first be able to release the emotions and thoughts that happen within their mind through their throat chakra.

If the person is unable to find a way to release all the emotions, they can become bottled up in the mind, polluting it in the process.

The throat chakra is your ability to express yourself, the feelings inside the heart, and the thoughts inside the mind.

It is located within your thought region, representing the color blue which is associated with healing, peace, calmness, and content.

When the throat chakra is balanced, you are able to speak freely without no one or nothing stopping or preventing you.

You are able to express yourself and who you truly are, saying whatever is on your mind.

Those who are able to express themselves are also able to inspire others around them by speaking up and sharing their own opinion.

You know that people listen to you and are able to understand you.

Not holding or suppressing emotions and thoughts back will be able to clear your mind, returning it to its 'pure' state.

Physically, the area of the throat is healthy and in balance with the rest of the body.

Both the mental and psychological aspect of one's life is also in balance.

The throat chakra is accountable for the maturity and development of your body, especially the mouth, jaws teeth, vocal cords, throat, nose, and voice.

Emotionally, this chakra is associated with self-expression, letting go of the feelings that you were holding up from past situations that left a mark on your heart and mind.

Letting go and expressing yourself can be done through crafting, music, writing, and in many other ways.

It is important to let go and share your feelings instead of bottling them up inside of you.

When the throat chakra is blocked, you will have trouble expressing what it is that you think and feel, this will turn you into an isolated and shy person.

Physically, the throat chakra causes problems within the endocrine system, the metabolic system, sore throats, the hormones in the body, and the thyroid gland.

This chakra also causes many diseases such as hypothyroidism, laryngitis, chronic throat defects, autoimmune thyroiditis, and many others relating to the body's growth and throat area.

When this chakra is out of balance emotionally, you will suffer from feelings of low self-esteem, restriction, low self-love, isolation, and no self-expression, as well as feeling like no one is here to listen to what you have to say.

This can cause depression and anxiety.

An underactive throat chakra revolves around insecurity, introversion, and timidity, meaning that when the throat is blocked, one will struggle with speaking up and sharing their opinion which will detach them from their true selves.

Other factors such as fear of speaking, introversion, and small voice are the causes of an underactive throat chakra.

If the throat chakra is overactive, one will find themselves experiencing a lack of control over their own speech, meaning they will talk too much and say whatever is on their mind without considering the consequences of their speech.

Those with an overactive throat chakra will experience talking too much, criticizing yourself and others, struggles in relationships and feeling like no one understands what they are saying.

Other factors such as gossiping, arrogance, rudeness, condescending, and overly criticality is caused by the overactive throat chakra.

Since the color blue is associated with the throat chakra, drinking plenty of water can help open and balance the throat chakra.

Especially drinking warm water or warm herbal tea which can help release tensions within the throat and clear out negative energies.

Singing your favorite songs or humming to a tune is also considered as a way of speaking, speaking can help awaken and balance the chakra as well as releasing any negative energies or tensions within that area.

It is also scientifically proven that singing can raise up one's mood, meaning it can help heighten your vibrations.

Specific yoga poses that involve you stretching the muscles can also help balance out not only the throat chakra but other chakras too.

Consider leaving some spare time out to practice different yoga poses that relate to different chakras, it will help ensure that your chakras will become balanced and healthy.

An open throat chakra will make you speak clearly and will help you express yourself more freely.

Meditation For The Throat Chakra

Comfort is key, it is important to get comfortable when meditating so both your mind and body can relax and not disturb you through this process.

Start your meditation by getting comfortable, sit down with your legs crossed, your spine straight and reaching out as high as possible.

Make sure your head is not sulking, but nice straight and tall.

Your head should face the front as the chin is raised, imagine as if you are balancing a book on your head.

Form a mudra with your hands, an 'okay' or 'zero' look-a-like sign by uniting the thumb and the index finger together before placing it on top of your knees, the palm of your hand facing upwards.

Begin by taking a few minutes to relax your body and muscles, focus your attention on your breathing as your chest rises and falls.

Breathe in deeply, inhale through your nose and hold the breath for up to three seconds before exhaling it through the mouth and dragging it out for another three seconds.

Make sure that when you are breathing in and out that you expand your chest, instead of breathing through your stomach.

When you are using the chest, the spine extends and moves along with the breathing, this will enable the relaxation found within the body, as well as the throat region.

Feel the way your lungs expand inside of you as they are filled with the air around you, cleansing you, and getting both your mind and body ready for the pure energy of your life force energy.

The throat region is often linked with your voice, in other words, the awakening of the throat chakra can be used to heal both.

The purpose of this meditation is to take your worries away from your inability to speak up so try not to let the feelings of worry and anxiety take over, this is your time to let go of all the bad thoughts and let you be the person you are meant to be as well as healing the throat and shoulder region.

Take a few minutes to simply relax your muscles and the body as you breathe in.

Bring your attention to your breathing as you inhale and exhale to help calm the mind.

Try your best to not listen to your thoughts and the mental clutter that is going on inside your head.

Instead, bring your focus to yourself as a being in this big universe.

Imagine yourself to be one with the universe as the energy flows through your body.

Don't think about anything else that you have to do or things that might be bothering, instead focus on breathing through your chest, making the lungs expand as you breathe in.

Relax the different parts of your body including your throat and neck.

As you breathe in, feel how the air comes through your nostrils, to your throat, and into your lungs before coming back up.

It is clearing all the negative energy out when you inhale and lets it all go as you exhale.

Breath in deeply, form a rhythm of your body.

Begin the usual energy harnessing by calling out to the Universe, and making an intention to harness your life force energy.

Imagine a white light emitting from within your body, spreading all throughout.

Allow for your mind's goals to be clear by setting an intention to receive healing within the throat area and helping yourself speak up more and become more involved with the community through the healing found within the chakra.

Focus on centering your energy within your hands. Imagine the white light surrounding you, traveling all the way to your hands.

Let the energy catch up and gather there, forming a bright ball of light.

Lift your hands up and place them on your collar bone, one hand over the other.

Visualize the healing energy leaving your hands and sinking deep through your body and making its way to the center of the throat chakra.

While allowing the pure white energy to settle down, begin to visualize the color blue, think of the first emotion or thing that pops into your head.

Feel your body calming down and becoming more stable.

Then picture that color blue evolving through your throat, a gently blue glow expanding every time you inhale, merging together with the energy of the white.

The throat chakra represents the gateway between the heart and mind, you are able to freely speak what is on your mind and in your heart.

But just by thinking about it can bring forth feelings of worry, so imagine all that worry resurfacing and letting it go as you breath out.

This is your voice and your own opinions, you have the right to express what is really in your heart.

This is also a perfect time to release any stress or worries that you might have by simply bringing them back up to the surface and making an intention for the bright blue light to simply purify them.

Let go of anything that might be bothering you.

Feel the tingling and warmth sensations through your neck as they emerge and push you to want to open your mouth and speak whatever is on your mind.

Bring an intention forward to receive a physical healing, through the healing of the mind.

Visualize that glow becoming bigger and brighter for three to five minutes before drawing your attention back to your breathing.

While still holding your hands on that area, use the mantra 'ham' which can create vibrations that have the power to alter the flow of energy within the communication center.

Once you spend at least two to three minutes healing that part of your body, move your hands upward and extend the healing energy to your throat.

Hold your hands there for another brief two to three minutes before rotating and moving them to the back of your neck.

Allow for the white energy to sunk in right around the throat while releasing blue energy of the throat chakra, bringing in healing and relaxation to that area.

Visualize the tensions going away, the muscles relaxing.

Hold your hands against your throat for a minute before moving down towards your shoulders.

Allow for the blue light to intervene with the white, creating a light blue hue.

Let that healing energy work its magic, traveling and releasing any negative tensions within the shoulder area.

Rest that energy against the shoulders for a brief minute.

Allow for the energy to evenly spread throughout your body, returning back to its original state, this time more powerful.

Imagine the body relaxing and energizing itself as your life force energy returns back throughout your body, purifying along the way.

Continue to deeply breathe in and out for about a minute, simply resting in the newfound sensation.

Slowly bring your attention to your body, the way you breathe, or the weight that your body holds against the earth below you.

Open your eyes. Remain seated in complete silence for another minute, allow for the healing energy to further settle in while you take some time to reflect on your meditation.

To finish off the treatment, tell someone what is on your mind or sing your favorite songs before carrying on with your day.

Speaking, reading or singing can help heal the throat region much faster after the chakra healing that you have experienced.

Chapter 8: The Third Eye Chakra

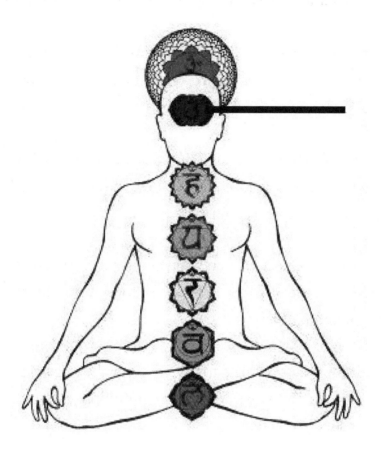

The sixth major chakra is the third eye chakra, it is also known as Anja which means 'beyond wisdom'.

Just like its translation, the third eye relates to the concept of following your gut feeling, intuition, and the discovery of psychic ability, all of which are able to abandon critical and logical thinking.

The third eye is also known as the sixth sense, it is able to see things that are far beyond what the human five senses notice.

With the third eye, one is able to see into different worlds and see into what people are feeling, something that the physical eyes can't do.

Spiritual gifts emerge through the opening of the third eye since the third eye is known to connect one to the spiritual world and set one on their spiritual journey.

The third eye is located in between one's eyebrows, usually in the middle of the forehead, it is known to be the origin of foresight and intuition.

The third eye is also linked to the color purple which is associated with inner wisdom, power, intuition, and extrasensory perception.

When the third eye chakra is in balance, one has the power to not only see into their own soul and look for what they desire but also look into other people's desires and motives.

It is very hard to trick one with an open and balanced third eye chakra, they are able to see through a person and recognize their true motives due to the heightened intuition ability.

You also achieve a sense of confidence within your life as well as the knowledge of what you are here for the sole purpose of living.

You will also gain a strong sense of inner truth and resolving physical problems that will happen in your environment will become a piece of cake due to your intuition which will guide you through your life.

Since the opening of the third eye grants the person different psychic abilities, it also enables easier communication between higher beings, angels, and spirits as well as seeing into the future and seeing your past lives.

Physically, the body is in great shape and is healthy, everything, as well as the flow of energy, is in balance.

Since the third eye is one of the strongest chakras found within the body, it also can strongly affect the chakras below it, opening and cleansing them, bringing equality within the body.

The area that the third eye is located will function better, eyesight can improve, the brain will receive more knowledge, and many other related functions will increase.

Emotionally, the one who has an open third eye chakra is able to live their life freely and control their emotions to not affect the environment.

Clear thinking, decision making, awareness, seeing past lies, spiritual gifts, and a stable mindset is all thanks to an open third eye.

However, when the third eye chakra is blocked, one will start to doubt their own existence.

The questions of what is the purpose of life will constantly cloud one's judgment, refraining them from living their life to the fullest.

You will become disconnected with yourself, your environment, and other people.

Physically, the third eye is responsible for the endocrine system which affects the person's growth, metabolism, and maturity, it is also responsible for the hormonal imbalance as well as the sleep cycle, fatigue within the body, migraines, and headaches.

Emotionally, the blocked third eye causes anxiety, an emotional imbalance, a lack of understanding of reality, depression, and a feeling of always being lost or lacking something.

An underactive third eye chakra can negatively affect one's thinking, how they process information, concentration, motivation, and inspiration.

You will also become fearful of the things that you do not understand or the unknown.

You may experience a lack of intuition, believing everything people tell you, live in constant fear, and low self-esteem.

An overactive third eye chakra is able to overindulgence your mind and your imagination.

One will constantly be in a daydreaming state, with no focus on what is happening right now in the present moment within their environment.

When the third eye is giving off too much energy, you will start to feel mentally exhausted, and overwhelmed.

You may experience anxiety, become judgemental, overly analytical, experience indecisiveness, clouded vision, and judgment.

Yoga can help open the third eye chakra, specific yoga poses such as the eagle pose and the child pose is programmed to help open and balance this chakra.

Exercising and eating healthy can help all the chakras be balanced due to the release of negative energies, however, specific foods that aid the third eye are foods with high omega-3 fats such as sardines, walnuts, chia seeds, and salmon can help enhance the third eye.

When opening your third eye chakra, you will enhance your intuition and creative inspiration.

Meditation For The Third Eye Chakra

Begin by selecting a place where you will feel comfortable and undisturbed, so lock your doors and turn off your phone.

Put on some loose clothing so you will feel more comfortable and lower the lights if they appear to be too bright for you.

It is recommended that you lay down during this process but you can sit up if you want to, however, you might find it hard to hold yourself upward in a chair.

When laying down, remember to not place a pillow under your head, only under your knees.

You can use a blanket to keep you warm but make sure to leave your hands by your sides on top of the blanket.

Proceed by slowly closing your eyes, breathing in deeply.

Focus on your breathing, in with the nose and out through the mouth.

Allow yourself to become in tune with the moment that is happening right now.

Feel your arms and legs become more relaxed.

Breathe in once again and this time hold the breath for an instant before you let go through your mouth, feel yourself relax even further.

Each time you breathe in or out, notice how every second your body becomes more and more relaxed.

Bring your attention to whatever is beneath you, if it's the bed or the ground, feel yourself connect to that energy.

Imagine your own energy connecting to the ground, like roots of a tree extending right into it, convincing and intertwining with the energy of the earth.

Embrace it and let it travel through your spine, let go of any anxiety, fear or resistance that you might have.

Allow for the earth's energy to travel upwards, all the way to the top of your head.

Imagine branches and leaves sprouting from the top of your head. You are a tree now, in your visualization.

You are one with the earth and the universe.

Allow for the energy to sprout and grow, for the roots to extend all the way below you and the branches and leaves to grow above you, reaching towards the ceiling.

Allow for your energy to resurface by visualizing a white light emerging from within your body.

Let that light grow, growing brighter with every breath you take.

Center your energy to your palms.

Close your eyes and concentrate on visualizing a white light emerging and entering your palms.

Let the energy rest there for a brief minute, gathering and forming a bright bulb of light. the third eye, immediately lifting your spirits up.

Focus on transmitting the energy and getting rid of any tensions and blockages.

Visualize the third eye-opening, enhancing your intuition and other psychic abilities.

Lift your hands up and place them on your head, each hand on the side of your temples.

Continue breathing deeply and slowly as you focus on releasing that energy into your mind with the intention to achieve healing.

Draw your attention to the middle of your eyebrows, where the third chakra is located.

Feel the energy that has emerged from your temples, making its way into the center of your forehead, feel the tingling as it is opening and radiating indigo light in all directions.

Visualize both lights combining together.

It small and faint at first but it is growing with each deep breath you take.

Let go of any uncertainties as you let the light evolve within your head, healing any tensed areas that you might have.

This experience is natural and completely safe.

Let the indigo light purify your frequency and heighten it, drawing positive feelings and experiences towards you.

Just relax, stay calm, breathe deeply and allow the experience to happen.

Let the indigo light open in your forehead, sending the gently streams of its like in all directions, relaxing you in the process.

You will start to feel the tingling sensations on that point if not already.

Enable to relax your body further and further.

Feel your weight on the floor or the mattress if you are laying down become lighter and lighter as more light flows around and through your body.

Allow your mind to open by itself naturally and on its own, don't force healing to happen otherwise too much energy can backfire and not work.

Let go of any thoughts or worries that can cloud your mind and stop you from continuing with the process.

Don't think too much of what can happen but relax your body further and focus on that warm, tingling sensation between your brows.

Using your index finger place the finger down on the third eye chakra and start to massage it in a clockwise circulation for women and an anticlockwise circulation for males.

Don't stop the light from flowing through your body as you massage your third eye, releasing its energy and letting it join together with the energy of the chakra.

Allow for yourself to feel the energy flow through you as your chakra point is opening.

Breath in deeply and out through your mouth to clear and cleanse any negative feelings or energy within your body, this is only a pure experience.

You might begin to see visions in your mind or hear something calling.

Since this healing practice is located so close to the third eye chakra, it will naturally begin to heal it and opening it.

The third eye is known to see things that can't be seen with your physical eyes, don't stress over the newfound feelings that might erupt in your body.

Simply continue this very pure experience.

It might begin to feel as if your mind just naturally wandered away, or you are having a daydream but you are not making it all up, that is the energy of the guides that are helping you realize what else needs to be done.

Begin to say the mantra 'Ksham' out loud for another two to three minutes to encourage the healing energy.

Slowly bring your attention to your breathing and make an intention for the energy to fall back evenly throughout your body, purifying and cleansing it in the process.

Make an intention to return your energy and spread it out evenly across your body.

Take some time to simply stay in the feeling of being aware and conscious of your surroundings but at the same time remind yourself of your pure intentions of healing and cleansing your body with the help of the third eye chakra.

When you feel as if you have meditated long enough and that you are done, slowly bring your consciousness back to what is happening right now.

Feel how heavy your body is becoming as you are focusing back on what is happening right now, in this present time.

Become aware of your legs, arms, hands, and body.

Open your mouth and say 'I am fully present, here and now'.

Your voice might come off as if you haven't spoken in a long time.

Take another and final deep breath, holding it in for a minute before slowly opening your eyes.

Take a minute to simply rest while reflecting on your meditation.

Chapter 9: The Crown Chakra

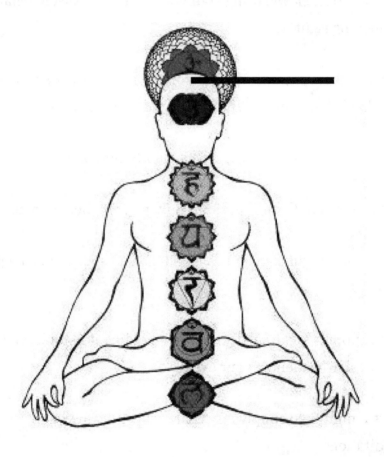

The last seventh chakra is known as the crown chakra, it is the hardest one to open and balance.

The crown chakra is also known as Sahasrara which translates to 'thousand-petaled'.

The crown chakra is the conscious chakra, compared to all the other chakras below it.

It revolves around your own personal consciousness and the subconscious part of the person.

This chakra is also responsible for attracting the same level of vibrational beings or things into one's life.

Located at the top of your head, the crown chakra acts like a magnet, pulling things the same vibrational frequency as your body towards you, it also extends upwards towards the universe and connects you to the higher energies.

The color this chakra is associated with indigo which represents devotion, inner wisdom, intuition, self-responsibility, spirituality, and trust.

When the crown chakra is in balance, you will feel a deep connection to the universe, the higher power, and with yourself.

You will also begin to feel as if something or someone is watching over you, making sure that you are going towards the right direction and clearing up your path towards success by making sure you avoid the difficulties and bad things in life, that is if you vibrate on a high level.

This energy is looking after you understand exactly what you desire and is able to help you achieve your goals along the way.

You will begin to feel a deep and strong sense of gratitude towards not only the universe but to yourself as well.

Feelings such as appreciation and love to yourself, your environment, and others around you will feel at peace surrounded by happiness and the feelings of safety.

When good things happen, they are able to affect our emotional states which affect the vibration level and works to attract more good things into our lives.

It is not only important to understand that even if bad things happen, but there is also always a good side to them, a hidden lesson that the universe is teaching you and it is up to you to be able to understand it and connect it to your life.

When this chakra is balanced, you will feel like everything within your life is going by perfectly and smoothly that is because you understand that you control your own life and can shape your own future with the power of thoughts and high vibrations.

There are absolutely no fears, worries, or problems resigning within your mind and even if there is one, you are able to deal with it on a positive level that doesn't even affect your wellbeing, either mentally, physically, emotionally, or spiritually.

Physically, the crown chakra is responsible for not only the mind area of the body but the other chakras too.

The mind is able to not only cause illnesses but heal them too.

When the mind is in balance with the body, the chakras can feel the peace and begin to open up their pure energies.

Emotionally, the crown chakra is aligned with the body, mind, and spirit and promotes a healthy mindset.

When the crown chakra is blocked, then it is able to influence and block other chakras due to this incredible amount of energy found within the crown.

You will begin to feel disconnected from the higher power as well as your spiritual journey.

You will feel as if there are no 'angels' watching over you and that your life is going downhill.

Physically, the body will begin to always feel exhausted, out of energy, minor headaches, trouble in many of the body's systems, organs, and glands.

Many parts of the body like the nervous system, brain, pituitary gland, and many others will be affected by the imbalance. Illnesses like

Illnesses such as brain tumors, amnesia, migraines, and cognitive delusions are caused by the imbalance within the crown chakra.

Emotionally, you will be filled with feelings of isolation, loneliness, insignificance, and a lack of connection.

The feelings of anxiety, stress, depression, hysteria, and other mental illnesses are all the causes of the crown chakra due to its location.

Not only that but negative thoughts and feelings are able to damage the body physically too when there is too much energy, especially negative energy, directed in a specific location, it can not only overflow but temporary stop that part of the body from working.

You will also constantly be afraid of change which can put you in an environment that will cause your unhappiness.

The underactive crown chakra is when the crown is blocked, thus blocking other chakras and the proper function of the body.

When it is underactive, it can limit one's ability to let go of either of the past or any materialistic needs.

It will detach you from the world around you and lead to s spiritual malaise.

Not only that but the relationships that you've built with other people will be strongly influenced the negative way.

Other signs of an underactive crown chakra are mental fog, feeling of greed, lack of motivation, and lack of inspiration.

An overactive crown chakra gathers way too much energy in one place, it can cause a disconnection of the physical body, as well as an overwhelmed feeling due to the energy.

This will affect the physical body, giving headaches and migraines.

Other signs such as superiority, lack of empathy, and a sense of elitism are all caused by the overactive crown chakra.

If you drink many herbal teas, they are guaranteed to help reduce the blockage within the crown chakra by clearing and cleansing the body from negative energy and toxins.

While consuming specific indigo-colored foods such as eggplants or grapes, they are known to help the crown chakra balance itself out.

Once your crown chakra is open, you will feel a spiritual awakening.

This chakra is a pathway to all the other chakras which is why it can be the hardest to open for some people.

Meditation For The Crown Chakra

Begin by getting comfortable by sitting with your legs crossed, spine straight and shoulders back.

Place your hands on top of your knees forming the mudra, an 'okay' or 'zero' look-a-like hand gesture by allowing the index and the thumb finger on each hand touch, or just simply place your palms on your knees, making them face upwards.

You can even meditate outside in nature which can help you feel more connected with the world around you.

Start off by simply breathing deeply, form a rhythm with your breath as you inhale and exhale.

Inhale through your nose, hold the breath anywhere from two to three seconds before letting go through your mouth.

Make sure when exhaling you drag the breath out for another two to three seconds.

Relax your body, each part at a time, like your legs, arms, belly, shoulders, etc.

If you find your mind drifting away, focus on your chest rising with each breath you take and the way it fills and expands your lungs with oxygen, this way your mind will become more relaxed and will prevent unnecessary thoughts from emerging when you get further into the meditation.

Once you feel as if your mind is settled in, then focus on feeling the energy through the ground with each breath you inhale, you can sense it more and more.

Continue by bringing up that energy, make it travel up your spine, through all of the previous regions with your body, purifying and relaxing on the way.

Let it travel up your spine and fill your other chakras in with energy and finally let it travel to the last region, the crown of your head, located slightly above your head.

It signifies your subconscious and conscious mind which can affect the body spiritually, physically, and mentally.

Let that energy gather around like a faint ball of light, floating just above your head.

With the color white to signify purity and spiritual awakening, let that light connect you to the universe.

Picture the bright glow becomes bigger and brighter with each deep breath that you inhale.

Spend some time focusing on this magnificent ball of energy and light, observe how it makes you feel emotionally and physically.

Can you feel overwhelming energy radiating from that ball of light?

Or can you feel tingling sensations or warmth coming from above that area?

At this point in the meditation, you might start to forget about your physical body as you are connecting with that energy on a spiritual level.

Surround yourself with that light, imagine it flowing through your head into your third chakra, then to your throat chakra and so on until it reaches your root chakra.

Let it rest at each point for a few seconds before moving on to the next chakra point.

Make the energy come back up to the crown at the top of your head.

Let it rest there for a few minutes, glowing and warming up your head before it comes back down to the root chakra and then back up to the crown once more.

The energy should travel up and down three times.

Let the energy flow back through your body to the ground through the bottom of your spine or where your body touches the ground.

Observe any emotions that you might be feeling when the energy was moving up and down or when it left and merged with the ground.

Breathe in deeply for a minute, resting in the sensation of having all your chakras united and opened.

Set an intention to resurface the energy that is already there within your body, ready to be called to healing.

Allow the bright light of your energy to resurface, surrounding your body like an auric field.

Let the light warm your body, purifying your soul and removing any negative impurities that are the cause of all of your troubles and pains.

Center all of that energy into the palms of your hands.

Allow the energy to form a ball of bright and pure light.

Lift your hands upright in front of your chest and form them into a Gassho position, the national praying and gratitude gesture.

Draw your life force energy further into your hands and ask the Universe for guidance to be able to heal your mind, getting rid of any bad habits that need to be healed.

Channel the energy in your hands.

Lift your hands up as high as you can while still maintaining the Gassho position.

Hold the position for a couple of seconds before lowering your hands and placing them one over the other on top of your head, where the crown is.

Feel the tingling sensations and make an intention to open this chakra.

Hold the position for about three minutes before beginning to massage your head with your hands in a circular clockwise motion.

Visualize giving more healing energy to the crown and your subconscious while concentrating on opening the crown and healing the mind, body, and soul.

Get rid of any negative emotions that do not belong within your mind by simply making at the intention for them to vanish.

Breathe in through your nose and out through your mouth.

Move your attention to your breathing and imagine that with every breath that you take, the air inside your lungs travels to all different parts of your body that the mind controls, purifying it and granting it the energy it needs to do its day to day activities.

Proceed to heal for another three minutes.

As the energy heals the body, keep on breathing deeply as you begin to lightly say the mantra 'ohm' to help further intensify the healing energy.

Proceed to carry your attention back to the top of your head before slightly moving your hands lower to your temples, engaging with the third eye region for a minute while stimulating the flow of energy.

Return the energy to all of the body, cleansing and purifying it with its powerful energy.

With your eyes still closed, take a deep breath, hold it for five seconds before letting it go with your mouth.

Give your chest the attention that it needs to ensure that the mind is aware of what is going on around it.

Take a minute to let the energy settle down as you meditate normally, keeping your mind from slipping away.

Slowly begin to bring your awareness back into your body by noticing the weight that you have against the physical world before you open your eyes and stay put for another minute.

When the crown chakra is being opened, you might feel like your head is going to explode.

You might get some headaches because the energies are being drawn to you and everything else that is not important is being let go.

When the energy is released, you will feel tingling sensations throughout your body, as well as heat, electricity, and sparks.

Raise your vibrations by doing something that you enjoy and love deeply after the meditation.

Consider taking some time off to relax while letting the energy that you just experienced settle in and continue healing you and the body.

Chapter 10: Yoga For Chakras

Each chakra also has a specific yoga pose that will help you awaken it, although it is recommended that when doing yoga, you should practice all the poses that you want by following a tutorial on how to do yoga and make up your own routine after a few practices.

Yoga or any form of exercise can help purify the body as well as your mind.

Yoga can help reduce stress, anxiety, depression, which are all causes of a blocked chakra.

Below are some easy yoga poses and their corresponding chakra points.

Root chakra:

Standing forward fold - Uttanasana (*ooh-tuhn-AHS-uh-nuh*)

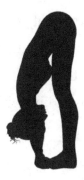

This pose is able to bring a sense of peace, harmony, and calmness to the mind.

The literal translation of its Sanskrit name is "intense stretch pose."

Instructions:

1. Begin with your hands on your hips.

2. Exhale as you bend forward at the hips, lengthening the front of your torso.

3. Bend your elbows and hold on to each elbow with the opposite hand.
   Let the crown of your head hang down.

   Press your heels into the floor as you lift your sit bones toward the ceiling. Turn the tops of your thighs slightly inward.

   Do not lock your knees.

4. If you can keep the front of your torso long and your knees straight, place your palms or fingertips on the floor beside your feet.
   Bring your fingertips in line with your toes and press your palms on the mat.

   Those with more flexibility can place their palms on the backs of their ankles.
5. Engage your quadriceps (the front thigh muscles) and draw them up toward the ceiling.
   The more you engage your quadriceps, the more your hamstrings (the rear thigh muscles) will release.
6. Bring your weight to the balls of your feet. Keep your hips aligned over your ankles.

7. Slightly lift and lengthen your torso with each inhalation.
   Release deeper into the pose with each exhalation.

   Let your head hang.
8. Hold the pose for up to one minute. To release, place your hands on your hips. Draw down through your tailbone and keep your back flat as you inhale and return to *Tadasana*. Repeat 5-10 times.

Garland pose - Malasana (*mah-LAHS-uh-nuh*)

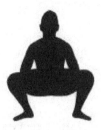

This yoga pose is perfect for bringing yourself closer to the earth's energies.

As you breathe slowly, you are able to quieten the mind.

Instructions

1. Begin by standing at the top of your mat with your arms at your sides.

    Step your feet about as wide as your mat.

2. Bend your knees and lower your hips, coming into a squat.

    Separate your thighs so they are slightly wider than your torso, but keep your feet as close together as possible.

If your heels lift, support them with a folded mat or blanket.

3. Drop your torso slightly forward and bring your upper arms to the inside of your knees.

   Press your elbows along the inside of your knees and bring your palms together in a prayer position.

   Work toward bringing your hands to your heart center and your forearms parallel to the floor.

4. Lift and lengthen your torso, keeping your spine straight and shoulders relaxed. Shift your weight slightly into your heels.

5. Hold for five breaths. To release, bring your fingertips to the floor. Then, slowly straighten your legs and come into Standing Forward Fold (*Uttanasana*).

Head to knee forward bend - Janu Sirsasana *(JAH-new shear-SHAHS-anna)*

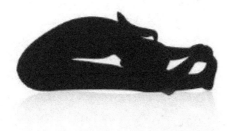

This pose brings a sense of grounding to the body and your energy while also developing flexibility in hips, hamstrings, and the back.

Instructions

1. Begin seated with both legs extended straight out in front of you, spine long.
2. Bend your right knee and bring the sole of your right foot to meet your inner left thigh.

   The outer (pinky toe) edge of your right foot should be on the ground, and the heel should be just in front of the groin.

3. Turn your torso to face the left foot.

Keep the left foot flexed and active, and energetically press down through the heel of the foot to engage the left leg.

4. On an inhale, extend both arms up alongside your ears.

    Reach your fingertips toward the ceiling and lengthen evenly along both sides of your body.

5. Maintaining the length along the spine, hinge at the hips on your next exhale and begin to fold forward over your extended leg.

    Let your hands fall wherever they may — the ground on either side of the extended leg, holding on to the calf, or perhaps even holding on to the left foot.

6. Avoid the tendency to collapse the chest and round the spine here in an effort to move deeper into your fold.

    Keep your shoulders back and relaxed away from your ears, broaden across the collarbones, and reach your sternum toward the toes of your left foot.

7. Remain in the pose for 5-10 deep breaths. On an inhale, make your way back to an upright position, switch your legs and repeat on the other side.

Sacral chakra:

Goddess Pose - Utkata Konasana" (*oot-KAH-tuh cone-AHS-uh-nuh*)

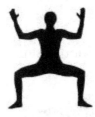

Good for generating emotional stability and creativity. This yoga pose corresponds with your sexual organs, reproductive system, fluidity, fertility, and creativity.

Instructions

1. From a standing position with the feet 3 feet apart, bend the elbows at shoulder height and turn the palms facing each other.

2. Turn the feet out 45 degrees facing the corners of the room, and as you exhale bend the knees over the toes squatting down.

3. Press the hips forward, press the knees back.

4. Drop the shoulders down and back and press the chest toward the front of the room.

5. Keep the arms active, as if they were holding a big ball over your head.

Look straight ahead with the chin parallel to the floor.

Dvipada pitham - Setu Bandhasana *(SET-too BAHN-dah)*

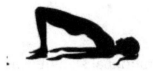

It provides a good stretch for your back muscles to help the healthy flow of energy.

Instructions

1. On the inhale gradually roll your hips up, pulling the knees slightly away from the hips, but making sure that the knees stay aligned over the ankles.

2. On the exhale roll down one vertebra at a time.

After repeating the pose few times hold the pose.

With every inhalation slightly lengthen from the neck to the knees, with every exhalation contract the abdomen and press your feet firmly into the ground. Keep the back of the neck long.

Solar plexus chakra:

Boat pose - Paripurna Navasana *(par-ee-POOR-nah nah-VAHS-anna)*

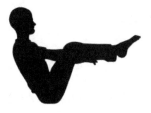

Great for fostering change and personal power into your life.

It helps you feel alive and promotes your self-esteem and confidence in order to make one take more action and become productive.

Instructions

1. Sit with your knees bent, feet on the floor.

Place your hands behind your knees, lift the chest, engaging the back muscles as you inhale

2. Engage your inner thighs and draw your lower belly in and up

3. Tip back on the back of your sitting bones and lift your feet up to about knee height, toes spread out

4. Bring your arms parallel to the floor

5. To go further, straighten your legs

6. Stay for 2-5 breaths, work up to 10 breaths

7. To come out of the pose, on an exhalation bring your feet down, and sit with a straight spine, holding on to your legs for a couple of breaths

Plank - Kumbhakasana (koom-bahk-AHS-uh-nuh)

This yoga pose has the ability to strengthen and heal the body by stirring up the solar plexus region.

It works by quickly building heat on the inside and outside of your body.

There are many variations for this yoga pose. In this case, we will do the one in the picture below.

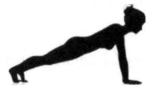

Instructions

- From all fours bring your shoulders over your wrists, fingers spread, middle finger pointing forward. Press your hands into the floor, firm the upper arms in towards each other.
- Draw the lower belly in and up.
- Extend one leg back with your toes tucked and then the other leg, so you are in a high push-up position. Your body is in a straight line from head to heels.
- Slide your shoulder blades down along the spine, firm them into the back and press the space between the shoulder blades up towards the ceiling.
- Engage your thigh muscles and lengthen the tailbone towards your heels.

- Keep pushing the floor away evenly with the palms of the hands and imagine you're pressing the heels back against a wall.

- Draw the legs together without actually moving them. This creates more core strength and stability.

- Look at the floor slightly forward, jaw relaxed. Breath is even and steady.

- You can stay in this pose anywhere between 5 breaths to a couple of minutes.

- To come out of the pose lower the knees to the floor.

Bow pose – Dhanurasana *(don-your-AHS-anna)*

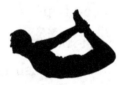

This yoga pose influences many important organs in the body such as the liver that is known to be the key organ for digestion.

It can also stimulate the blood flow and the energy flow within the body.

Instructions

1. Begin by lying flat on your stomach with your chin on the mat and your hands resting at your sides.

2. On an exhalation, bend your knees. Bring your heels as close as you can to your buttocks, keeping your knees hip-distance apart.

3. Reach back with both hands and hold onto your outer ankles.

4. On an inhalation, lift your heels up toward the ceiling, drawing your thighs up and off the mat.

   Your head, chest, and upper torso will also lift off the mat.

   Draw your tailbone down firmly into the floor, while you simultaneously lift your heels and thighs even higher.

   Lift your chest and press your shoulder blades firmly into your upper back.

   Draw your shoulders away from your ears.

5. Gaze forward and breathe softly. Your breath will become shallow, but do not hold your breath.

6. Hold for up to 30 seconds.

7. To release, exhale and gently lower your thighs to the mat.

Slowly release your legs and feet to the floor.

Place your right ear on the mat and relax your arms at your sides for a few breaths. Repeat the pose for the same amount of time, then rest with your left ear on the mat.

Heart chakra:

<u>**Camel pose**</u> - Ustrasana *(oosh-TRAHS-anna)*

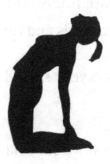

It is good for being more empathetic, joyful, and loving.

It helps awaken the power of unconditional love inside of you through acceptance, compassion, and forgiveness.

Instructions

1. Kneel with the body upright and hips stacked over the knees. Take a blanket or fold your mat under your knees if they are sensitive.

2. Draw your hands up the side of your body until your thumbs reach your armpits.

   Hook your thumbs into your pits for support as you start to open your chest toward the ceiling.

3. Maintain the position of your chest as you reach your hands back one at a time to grasp your heels.

   If you need a little more height, tuck your toes under. Otherwise, the tops of the feet can be flat on the floor.

4. Bring your hips forward so that they stay over your knees.

5. If it feels good, let your head come back, opening your throat.

   If that doesn't work for your neck, you can keep the chin tucked instead.

6. Release by bringing your chin toward your chest and hands to your hips.

Firm your abs and support your lower back with your hands as you slowly bring your body to an upright kneeling position.

<u>Bridge pose</u> - Setu Bandha Sarvangasana *(SAY-too BAHN-duh shar-vahn-GAHS-uh-nuh)*

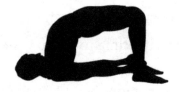

This pose is a gentler version of the Wheel Pose.

It can help create flexibility and strength within your spine.

Perform this pose if the Wheel pose is more difficult.

<u>Instructions</u>

1. Begin lying comfortably on your back in a supine position.

Allow the back of your head and the backs of your shoulders to rest on the ground, and avoid moving your head from side to side as you enter this pose to protect your neck.

2. Bend your knees and place the soles of your feet flat down on your mat.

   Ensure that the feet are parallel and separated about hip-distance apart and that your weight is distributed evenly across the soles of both feet.

3. Walk your feet in towards you until you can just graze your heels with your fingertips.

   Root your feet down strongly into the ground.

4. On an inhale, lift your hips up high toward the ceiling and begin to walk your shoulders underneath you.

   Interlace your fingers and press your forearms down into the mat to get more lift in the hips.

5. Note the tendency for the knees to want to splay apart as the hips lift higher and firm up through the inner thighs without gripping the buttocks.

Squeezing a block between the knees can be helpful to keep the thighs hip distance apart and parallel here.

6. Continue to refine the pose by moving your chest towards your chin (not chin to chest!), lengthening your tailbone towards your feet, and perhaps most importantly, relaxing your face.
7. Hold the pose for 5 full, deep breaths.
8. On an exhale, release the clasp of your hands, begin to walk your shoulders out from underneath you, and slowly roll down onto the ground, one vertebra at a time.

Feel free to bend your knees into your chest and wrap your arms around your legs for a well-deserved hug.

<u>Upward facing dog pose</u> - Urdhva Mukha Shvanasana
(OORD-vah MOO-kah shvon-AHS-anna)

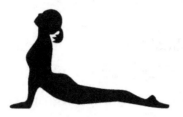

This yoga pose can help strengthen and tone your spine and arms as well as making your body more flexible.

This pose is recommended for those who always use computers for their work to help relieve any tensions.

Instructions

1. Begin lying on your belly with your legs extended straight back behind you and the tops of your feet relaxed down on the mat, hip-distance apart.
2. Plant your palms beside your ribs so that your elbows are bent approximately 90 degrees and your forearms are relatively perpendicular to the floor.
3. On an inhale, press firmly into your palms and straighten your arms, lifting your torso, hips, and the tops of your thighs up off the ground.

The shoulders should be stacked directly over the wrists and the creases of the elbows should face forward.

4. Relax your shoulders away from your ears, then begin to roll your shoulders back and find the action of pulling your chest forward through your upper arms.

    Keep the chin in line with the floor or lifted slightly, avoiding the urge to crank the head back in order to send the gaze up to the ceiling (which can compress the back of the neck).

5. Continue to refine the pose by firming your thighs and upper outer arms and drawing your low belly in toward your spine.

    Remain for 5-10 deep breaths before transitioning to Downward-Facing Dog or lowering back down onto the belly.

Throat chakra:

Supported shoulder stand - Salamba Sarvangasana *(sah-LOM-bah sar-van-GAHS-anna)*

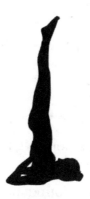

Great for when you want to become more outspoken and are looking to find your own voice.

This pose helps by relaxing the shoulder and neck muscles and releasing it from any tensions.

Instructions

1. Begin by lying flat on your back with your legs extended and your arms at your sides, palms down.

   Bend your knees and place the soles of your feet flat on the floor.

2. On an inhalation, use your abdominal muscles to lift your legs and hips off the floor. Curl your torso and bring your knees in toward your face.

   Then, lift your hips and bring your torso perpendicular to the floor.

3. Bend your elbows and place your hands on your lower back with your fingertips pointing up toward the ceiling.

   Keep your elbows on the ground, shoulder-width apart. Do not let your elbows splay out to the sides.

4. When you are comfortable, lift your thighs so they are vertical to the floor, keeping your knees bent.

   Draw your tailbone toward your pubic bone.

   Then, straighten your legs fully and reach your feet up to the ceiling. Lift through the balls of your feet.

5. Try to bring your shoulders, hips, and feet into one line.
6. Keep your head and neck in line with your spine and do not turn your head.

   Draw your shoulder blades firmly into your upper back.

   Keep a space between your chin and chest, and soften your throat.

Gaze toward your chest.

7. Hold the pose for 10-25 breaths.

More advanced practitioners can hold the pose for five minutes or longer. To release the pose, slowly lower your feet back to the ground.

Fish pose Matsyasana *(mot-see-AHS-anna)*

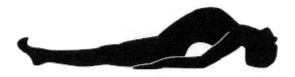

It stretches the back muscles, the shoulders, and the neck region.

Instructions

1. Begin by lying on your back with your legs extended and your arms resting alongside your body, palms down.

2. Press your forearms and elbows into the floor and lift your chest to create an arch in your upper back.

   Lift your shoulder blades and upper torso off the floor.

   Tilt your head back and bring the crown of your head to the floor.

3. Keep pressing through your hands and forearms.

   There should be very little weight pressing through your head.

4. Keep your thighs active and energized.

   Press outward through your heels.

5. Hold for five breaths.

To release the pose, press firmly through your forearms to slightly lift your head off the floor.

Then exhale as you lower your torso and head to the floor.

Third eye chakra:

Easy pose - Sukhasana *(soo-KAHS-uh-nuh)*

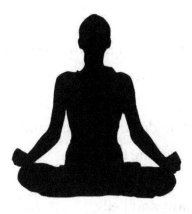

Good for wanting to learn new things and learning to trust your own instincts.

This pose is associated with awakening your sixth sense and intuition.

It is the universal meditational pose that strengthens the back and promotes a healthy flow of energy from the crown to the root chakra, passing all the other chakras, and awakening them.

Instructions

1. Come into a seated position with the buttocks on the floor, then cross the legs, placing the feet directly below the knees.

Rest the hands on the knees or the lap with the palms facing up or down.

2. Press the hip bones down into the floor and reach the crown of the head up to lengthen the spine.

    Drop the shoulders down and back, and press the chest towards the front of the room.

3. Relax the face, jaw, and belly.

    Let the tongue rest on the roof of the mouth, just behind the front teeth.

4. Breathe deeply through the nose down into the belly.

    Hold as long as comfortable.

5. Release and change the cross of your legs.

Child's pose – Balasana *(bah-LAHS-anna)*

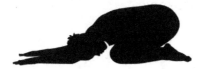

When performing this pose, make sure that you connect your forehead to the earth below you, it will create light pressure and stimulate the opening of the third eye with the help of the earth's energies.

Instructions

1. Starting on your knees, sit back on your heels.
2. Inhale lengthen through the spine.
3. Exhale as you walk your arms in front of you, bringing your torso down so that you can rest your forehead on the mat.
4. Rest your arms by your sides with your palms facing up near your feet.
5. Breathe deeply for as long as you like. This pose should feel completely relaxing.

Crown chakra:

<u>Tree pose:</u> - Vrikshasana (vrik-SHAH-suh-nuh)

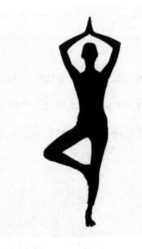

This pose is associated with feelings of guardedness, stableness, survival, calmness, harmony, nature, and the earth's energy.

It can help form a connection with the universe.

<u>Instructions</u>

1.   Begin with your arms at your sides.

Distribute your weight evenly across both feet, grounding down equally through your inner ankles, outer ankles, big toes, and baby toes.

2. Shift your weight to your left foot. Bend your right knee, then reach down and clasp your right inner ankle.

    Use your hand to draw your right foot alongside your inner left thigh.

    Do not rest your foot against your knee, only above or below it.

    Adjust your position so the center of your pelvis is directly over your left foot.

    Then, adjust your hips so your right hip and left hip are aligned.

3. Rest your hands on your hips and lengthen your tailbone toward the floor.

    Then, press your palms together in prayer position at your chest, with your thumbs resting on your sternum.

4. Fix your gaze gently on one, unmoving point in front of you.

5. Draw down through your left foot.

Press your right foot into your left thigh, while pressing your thigh equally against your foot.

6. Inhale as you extend your arms overhead, reaching your fingertips to the sky.

   Rotate your palms inward to face each other.

   If your shoulders are more flexible, you can press your palms together in prayer position, overhead.

7. Hold for up to one minute.

   To release the pose, step back into Mountain Pose.

   Repeat for the same amount of time on the opposite side.

Easy pose - - Sukhasana *(soo-KAHS-uh-nuh)*

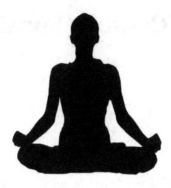

This universe meditational pose can also be used for the crown chakra due to its power to awaken the intuitive side of yourself.

This intuition can help you gain more insight as to what more is needed to be completed or done to awaken this chakra.

It can also help access any messages from the universe and the higher power.

It promotes a healthy flow of energy that is able to awaken all the other chakras.

Chapter 11: Crystals For Chakras

Another effective method when it comes to unblocking chakras, balancing them, and getting rid of any negative energies is with crystals.

Crystals have been around for thousands of years, many even believe they might just be as old as time itself.

Crystals can be used for many different purposes such as healing the body, manifesting abundance, attracting love, and most importantly balancing the chakras.

Simply by directing your energy as well as setting your intentions into the crystal that is best associated with the specific chakra that you are trying to awaken, you will be able to change your life, provide protection, boost one's energies, achieve your goals, and promote your health.

Each crystal and stone that you come across has a different use and meaning to them as well as specific diseases that it is able to heal, either physical or mental ones.

There are many benefits that all crystals share in common such as boosting energy.

All crystals are able to boost the energy within the body which is required to help heal and achieve specific goals.

Not only do crystals boost the energy, but they also cleanse, and purify it at the same time.

Since the main cause of blocked chakras is the toxic energy flow, having crystals around us constantly will help cleanse the energy and the chakra centers at the same time.

However, there are some basic things you should know about crystals before you jump into healing.

Crystals not only pick up the vibrations of other beings, but some of them might even have greater energies absorbed within.

Many people in the past decades believed that the gemstones were corrupted by the sins of Adam from the story of Adam and Eve.

It was said that the crystals could potentially be occupied by evil entities, it was also believed that the crystal's magical properties would fade if the crystal was handed over to a sinner.

This is where the belied of charging and cleansing the crystals originated from.

This is also why many crystals must be blessed, prayed upon, or cleansed especially before wearing or carrying any crystals.

If one forgets to cleanse the crystal, then the crystal can attract negative, low vibrational problems or low vibrational people into the life of the one who carries or wears the crystal.

All crystals once bought from the store need to be cleansed.

Crystals work to absorb negativity and pick up lower vibrations, this often 'fills' up the crystal and makes it work less efficient.

In order to recharge the crystal and bring it back to its full power, simply cleanse it the very day you get it.

Selenite is one of the only crystals that doesn't require to be cleansed, in fact, it works wonderfully to cleanse and charge surrounding crystals.

This crystal is definitely a must-have!

Simply leave your brand new crystals next to Selenite overnight and you will feel the energy of the crystals being restored back to its high frequency.

Another method is to wait until the moon is full and leave the crystal on the window still under the moonlight.

The full moon works by purifying and charging the crystal, restoring and returning back all the magical properties.

On the night of the full moon, leave your crystal outside on the balcony, if you don't have a balcony then use a windowsill.

The crystal will absorb the pure energy of the moon once exposed to direct moonlight.

Another easier way is to make moon water.

Moon water is simply water left under the full moon, the water absorbs the energy of the full moon and can be used any time as long as it is not exposed to sunlight.

Once you obtain the moon water, you can use it to charge your crystals any time you like, without needing to wait for the full moon.

Simply rub some water on the crystals and leave it to dry.

The moon water can also be used to charge candles and cleanse the home environment.

The last technique is by leaving the crystal exposed to sunlight for a few hours can also cleanse it.

The sun has powerful energy and is associated with the element of fire, one of the strongest elements out of the four.

Simply place your crystal on a windowsill and leave it for at least one hour, make sure you do not overexpose the crystal.

The sun doesn't just cleanse the crystal, it charges it too.

You might feel overwhelmed by the energy collected within that crystal when you start to do your healing work with it.

Too much energy used for healing can lead to some unpleasant side effects.

When starting off and using any crystal healing techniques, make sure that the crystal or crystals that you are planning on using have been cleaned properly to ensure that you will receive the positive energy and vibrations within, it also is responsible for making sure that one doesn't worsen their condition.

When it comes to healing with crystals, there is no such thing as right or wrong healing practice.

It all comes down to connecting with the crystal by holding it in your hand, meditating with it for a few minutes, and setting your intentions and projecting them into the crystal.

As long as the intentions match the vibrations of the crystal's properties then the healing practice will be successful.

However, many of those who use crystals for healing like to use more than one in order to amplify the energy within the practice.

One cannot simply hold all the crystals in their hands while each of their vibrations intercepts with each other, this will simply mess up the healing practice since each crystal has its own different properties.

This is where the concept of crystal grids come in.

Crystal grids are patters that are used when multiple crystals are needed to heal the mind, body, soul, or even restore one's energy.

They are designed to amplify one's intention for a successful crystal healing and make it more effective.

The crystals that are used within the crystal grid relate to one's intentions and are used to amplify the purpose for this crystal healing.

Different shapes and colors of crystals also play an important role in the energy that is harnessed during the practice.

The crystal grid designs are usually based on sacred geometry, they are designed for any purpose.

When crystals are arranged properly, their energies support one another and even increase.

This is why the intention of the crystal healing needs to be specified before starting the crystal grid.

There are many different purposes in which the crystal grids are used for.

Mainly they are used for protection, healing, love, and manifestation.

They work by harnessing the energy of the surrounding crystals, combining it, and creating a sort of shift within that energy which can be used to bring the desired change.

There are no specific rules when it comes to crystal grid except following your own intuition.

It is best to listen to what your Higher Self is telling you and the best way to accomplish that is by following what you think is best.

Of course, there a crystal grid templates but making your own crystal grid just magnifies the energy used.

Many people use a piece of paper or cloth to draw a sacred geometry, there are also many that can be bought and found online for free.

Crystals for the Root Chakra:

Garnet is the to-go crystal when it comes to healing the root chakra.

Garnet is associated with inspiration, sensuality, positive thinking, passion, success, romantic love, inspiration, and self-confidence.

It is known as an energy stone that revolves around re-energizing the root chakra and cleansing it.

It can promote a smoother flow of energy not just within the root, but the surrounding chakras too.

Balancing and purifying has never been easier with the help of garnet which works by bringing passion and serenity into the mind and body.

Another crystal that is associated with the root chakra is **carnelian**.

A red carnelian can help keep the healing energy and vibrations close to your root chakra, affecting it in a positive way.

It will ensure that the root is being cleansed, balanced, and active throughout the day.

Carnelian is able to bring appreciation, courage, higher self-esteem, a better memory, individuality, and harmony to those who use the crystal.

It is best known to be a stabilizing stone that can help restore the balance within the root.

This crystal can also help restore motivation, promote positive thinking, dispel apathy, creativity, vitality, and fill one will inspirations.

Black tourmaline is another good crystal for the root chakra healing.

It is a protective stone that works by repealing the negative energies and psychic attacks that are directed to wherever the stone is located.

Many people choose to wear this stone because of that, however, it has other good qualities such as cleansing and purifying the root chakra.

It transforms and brings negative energy into the light, heightening the vibration and turning it into something good.

Lastly, the **tiger's eye crystal** is mostly used to empower the root chakra.

This can help speed up the process of healing that it undergoes.

It is associated with confidence, courage, finding true desires, discovering the purpose of life, easing the feelings of worry or fear, and grounding the user.

It further deepens the understanding of your own true desires while giving inspiring vibrations to help stabilize the energy of the root chakra.

Tiger's eye can also help one see the situation from a different perspective which can eliminate feelings of anxiety and fear.

Crystals for the Sacral Chakra:

A perfect crystal for the sacral chakra is the **orange carnelian** which is also a healing crystal.

It helps heal, clear, and balance this chakra along with the other surrounding chakras such as the root and the solar plexus.

It can also boost your intuition, and energize the body.

This crystal can also be used to balance the root chakra too.

If you choose to use the same crystal for different chakras, make sure that you set your intentions straight to not mistake the energy that the crystal will harness.

A **brown colored tiger's eye** is well suited when it comes to activating and balancing the sacral chakra.

This crystal balances the physical, emotional, and spiritual aspects of a person while also healing any illnesses and diseases.

Tiger's eye is an energy stone, it works perfectly by cleansing the energy within the body and activating the proper flow of Ki which can get rid of tiredness and exhaustion within the body.

Spessartine garnet can also be used on the sacral chakra.

It works by stimulating the inspiration, sexuality, and creativity within your body in order to heighten the connection to your life and in order to feel more alive.

This stone is known to hold a lot of energy, one should always be precautious when interacting with this stone.

Make sure that you only be exposed to its energy at least a couple of minutes a day until your tolerance will heighten otherwise you will begin to feel weak and sick due to the overwhelming amount of energy.

This crystal also enhances the rational mind, analytical process, and encourages you to take action towards your goals.

Crystals for the Solar Plexus Chakra:

Peridot is one of the main crystals that are used on the solar plexus.

It's main use it to cleanse and activate this chakra.

It works as a powerful cleanser alleviating many negative feelings such as bitterness, greed, hatred, irritation, and jealousy.

It can also neutralize the toxins within the body before releasing them, this is why it is good for the solar plexus.

Since this chakra is emotionally related, releasing foul emotions such as anger, guilt, and stress.

This crystal is also able to help open up the heart to good emotions like happiness by enhancing one's relationships with people through granting confidence, motivations, and assertion.

When activating the solar plexus chakra, you need to start off your cleansing process within any physical contact if you are working with other chakras.

Peridot can also be used to open the heart chakra.

As a necklace, peridot can help prevent any negative energies influencing your awakening and healing process by wearing it around your neck.

This is especially useful when you have awakened all of your chakras and are undergoing the healing process.

Golden-Yellow colored labradorite is best known to be a sunstone or a bytownite.

This crystal is useful when one is undergoing change, perseverance, and even imparting strengths.

It is known to balance and protect the aura within the body as well as ground the spiritual energies and raise one's awareness of the world around them.

Labradorite can also promote psychic abilities and even strengthen your intuition.

When used on the solar plexus, it can help enhance your confidence, vitality, and assertiveness which are the main three emotions needed to balance out this chakra.

This stone also brings positive transformation.

Citrine is yet another great healing stone for the solar plexus.

It is known to impact one's mood drastically bringing emotions such as enthusiasm, wonder, delight, and joy.

When it comes to the solar plexus chakra, this crystal works to open, cleanse, and activate the chakra through energizing the body.

When a lot of energy is required, this stone stimulates the life force energy which aids in the proper functions of the body, opens intuition, draws wealth, promotes abundance, and brings prosperity to the carrier of the citrine crystal.

The **tiger's eye** is probably one of the most powerful solar plexus crystal that is used for healing.

Specifically golden-brown in color, this stone can help the solar chakra function properly as well as creating a well-balanced and empowered body, mind, soul, and environment.

Crystals for the Heart Chakra:

Rose Quartz is known as the crystal of love and peace.

It is also one of the few crystals that specialize in the balance and opening of the heart chakra due to its strong positive energy.

Love is known as the go-to when raising vibrations due to the pure energy that resigns within.

This crystal is very warm, gentle, and filled with nourishing energy that works to deepen the feelings that the heart has, as well as increasing the energy of unconditional love.

It can help relax the muscles, stay in the moment, and bring smooth and peaceful healing energy to the body, mind, and soul.

When it comes to the heart chakra, the rose quartz gives love to the body and mind, it also grants better judgment, mental clarity, and an open mindset when it comes to relationships and feelings.

This crystal has high energy that it is possible for anyone to feel its vibrations, even if they vibrate on a low level.

Aquamarine is another crystal that has the healing properties to heal the heart chakra through cleansing, soothing, and activating it.

It works by purifying the body and the flow of Ki.

It is associated with the sea and the water which means it can also be used on the throat chakra.

This calming and soothing crystal can help inspire the truth, let go of the past, heal the emotions, and grant trust.

When using this stone, make sure that you do not exceed the limit of five to ten minutes of contact in your first couple of tries.

Aquamarine has very strong energy, it may feel overwhelming at times if used for a long period of time when one's body is not used to the high energies.

Peridot, either a pale green or an olive-colored, works perfectly when it comes to opening and balancing the heart chakra.

This crystal restores the balance of energies within the body, mind, and soul while promoting peace, harmony, mental clarity, and better judgment.

It is a healing crystal for the heart and can be used to heal from grief after losing a friend or a partner.

This crystal is also able to mend relationships or attract new ones into your life.

Green aventurine has also a very soothing effect on the body once used to heal.

This crystal aims to promote harmony and balance within the body as well as improve any romantic or personal relationships.

Crystals for the Throat Chakra:

Lapis Lazuli is one of the main crystals that have the energy to balance and heal the throat chakra.

Lapis Lazuli, especially a bluish-white or blue color works by expanding the auric field that is used to protect the body from any negative energy while the chakra undergoes its healing process.

Lapis lazuli can give one strength to help overcome the blockage that is stopping one from speaking up as well as repair the inner voice of the one who uses the crystal.

Wearing lapis lazuli as a necklace or earrings can help benefit the throat chakra and the third eye chakra, promoting the healing process and always protecting the body.

Moonstones are also able to help the throat chakra.

They are associated with the mother moon which represents deep healing, water, and the sacred female energies.

This crystal is able to bring you back to wholeness, make you more aware of its nourishing and deeply feminine energy.

It also takes its time to heal the throat to ensure that the process will be effective.

Moonstones can also help cleanse and heal other surrounding chakras as well.

Dark blue iridescent labradorite crystals are used to increase the energy within the throat chakra to ensure its healing.

It is also used to increase the energies of other crystals which is why it is rarely used alone.

Labradorite enhances strength and perseverance which is what is needed to ensure the opening of the throat chakra.

Since this chakra is more mentally connected, it grants light to the human soul, ensuring that everything will be okay.

Its high vibrational crystal is mostly worn as an earring or a necklace used along with one other relating crystal.

Amazonite, one that is bluish-green or simply green, can also be used to heal the throat chakra.

Amazonite helps the person not only be able to overcome what is holding them back but also see both sides of the problem before making their judgment.

It specializes in soothing emotional traumas and getting rid of emotions such as fear and worry.

This crystal calms the nervous system and the brain in order to balance out the physical, emotional, and mental aspects of a person.

It also balances the masculine and feminine energies.

It falls at the right pace in order to open the throat chakra, not rushing it but taking its time to ensure that through the process one is healed effectively.

Crystals for the Third Eye Chakra:

Sodalite contains a high amount of salt which is why it is mainly used to cleanse and get rid of negative energies that block the third eye from activating and granting you its benefits.

This crystal specializes in cleansing by getting rid of the toxins not only within the mind but the body too, which is why it is able to encourage a healthy flow of Ki that can be used to open the other chakras.

It can also help enhance creativity, promote mental clarity, inspiration, and grant clear communication to those who possess the crystal.

Sodalite can also help one think more logically and clearly when it gets rid of negativity and expands the space for positivity and inner peace.

Lapis Lazuli can help with the opening of the third eye chakra.

This marbled blue-colored crystal is associated with awareness and self-expression, because of this, it gives the crystal a boost when it comes to spiritual transformation and enlightenment which is what the third eye chakra is all about.

It is able to bring inner peace to the mind, and balance out all of the energies within the body.

It especially eliminates negative thoughts since the third eye is located within the mind.

Labradorite has very powerful energy which is why if used, one should be cautious.

It is an energizing stone that stimulates the flow of energy within the third eye region.

This will help to open and clean that area.

You may also place this stone under your pillow in order for the healing energies to continue healing your third eye even when you are deep in sleep.

Amethyst can also help heal the third eye chakra by opening and cleansing the region.

It grants the energy of passion and fire as well as sobriety, temperance, creativity, and spirituality.

It works by eliminating the negative energy within the body, replacing it with positivity which heals the imbalance found within the third eye chakra.

When using this crystal, you can wear it as an earring so it will be always on you and close to the region of the third eye.

It can also help protect you during your healing process.

Crystals for the Crown Chakra:

Clear Quartz is best known for its power as a healing stone for the crown chakra.

This crystal works by balancing and cleansing the area, stabilizing and aligning the other six chakras while the crown chakra is being activated.

It gets rid of any unwanted energy within the body, freeing up the space for positivity and good energy.

It can also help increase the harmony within the body, bring peace to the mind, and balance your entire being.

When using the clear quartz to open the crown chakra and balance the other six chakras, the energy flows downwards when opened, cleansing out the other six areas found inside the body.

Each chakra helps one and another to promote the healthy flow of energy.

Black tourmaline is a grounding stone that possesses healing properties for the crown chakra.

It increases the effectiveness of the crown chakra's opening.

It also helps the healing process by blocking out any negative energies that would want to interfere with the healing.

Chapter 12: Affirmation For Chakras

Since each chakra is responsible for a specific region within the body, it is also responsible for our feelings and emotions.

For example, the root chakra gives one the feeling of security and safety while the sacral chakra is about your enjoyment of the life around you.

So when chakras are blocked, the thoughts and emotions are affected.

Thoughts and feelings are also able to affect chakras too.

When thinking negatively and always worrying about the world around you, you are closing off your own chakras.

If you change the way that you think, you are able to change your actions and influence your life for the better.

Saying affirmations can change the way that you think, but only if you let yourself believe it rather than say the affirmations but complain for the rest of the day.

Training your mind to think positively can bring good change into your life, but this means reprogramming your mind and not just by saying a couple of words, you got to put your feelings into it too.

Being able to feel and believe what you are telling yourself is how you will be able to retrain your mind.

If you simply say the words and go forth about your day without thinking about them or acting like what you said to yourself, then those words have no context and no meaning behind them.

There are simply just words.

It will take so much longer if you don't put your heart and soul into it.

Affirmations are only made easy if you choose to believe in those words, believe in change, and in yourself.

Saying and feeling the affirmations are only part of the process.

They are like a seed within the soil that you need to constantly water for it to grow.

Watering the seed is like adding onto your words within your life.

You are building up towards that affirmation.

For example, if your affirmation was something to do with your confidence in yourself then you would not only go forth about your day thinking confidently, but you got to put a bit of work too, you got to act confident.

This is how change happens.

Affirmations work by strengthening and healing any part of your life, but it is also up to you to help along that process for it to be more effective and work at a faster pace.

When working with chakras, you are bringing attention to that part of your emotions or thoughts that you wish to change, you are granting that chakra focus and attention, and only the good kind of energy.

Eventually, the chakra begins to open as you take on that form of a confident individual that you only wished you'd be.

You have to believe in your affirmations and in yourself before you can expect to open your chakras.

Make a habit of repeating to yourself an affirmation when you wake up, first thing in the morning to set your mind into the right mindset and to know your goals for the day.

Root Chakra Affirmations:

"I am enough as I am."

"I am in touch with the earth and the universe"

"I am always safe and happy"

"I love myself and my body"

"My future is financially secure and I have nothing to worry about"

"I am open to change"

Sacral Chakra Affirmations:

"I embrace my sexuality"

"I am beautiful and happy the way that I am"

"I am comfortable in my own skin"

"I am safe"

"I am open to expressing myself in creative ways"

"I am deeply connected with my soul"

Solar Plexus Chakra Affirmations:

"I am beautiful and confident"

"I can achieve anything I set my mind to"

"My body is healthy and strong"

"I feel motivated to pursue my dreams"

"I understand that everything is a lesson to my spiritual journey"

"I value myself"

Heart Chakra Affirmations:

"I love myself for who I am"

"I embrace the love for myself"

"I am open to new and healthy relationships"

"I am able to give and receive love"

"I am grateful for everything that I have"

Throat Chakra Affirmations:

"My thoughts are positive"

"I am able to express myself positively, clearly, and truthfully"

"I think before I speak"

"I am able to say 'no' when I want to"

"Everyone listens to what I have to say"

"I listen to my heart"

Third Eye Chakra Affirmations:

"I understand the lesson behind the situations in my life"

"I trust my intuition"

"I can see the deeper truths and connections in life"

"My third eye is open"

"I am connected to the universe"

"I let my intuition guide me"

Crown Chakra Affirmations:

"I understand and I know"

"I feel a connection with other beings"

"I am one with the universe"

"I understand the deeper meaning behind everything"

"I experience love, joy, and peace in my life"

"I am light, I am love and I am joy"

"I have a high frequency and vibration"

Conclusion

Thank you for making it through to the end of *Chakra Healing For Beginners* let's hope it was informative and able to provide you with all the tools you need to achieve your goal of awakening your chakra points.

The next step is to put everything you learned to the test, start meditating and changing your life step by step.

Awakening and opening your chakras might take a while, but with a lot of practice and willpower, you will achieve your goal.

With the help of your open chakras, you will be able to harness their energy and help heal your body, mind, and soul.

Every little challenge life throws at you is just an obstacle for you to overcome in order to achieve success in your life.

Thank you for reading and good luck on your journey!

Finally, if you find this book useful in any way, a review on Amazon is always appreciated!

CPSIA information can be obtained
at www.ICGtesting.com
Printed in the USA
BVHW041104130421
604816BV00001B/500

9 781801 875714